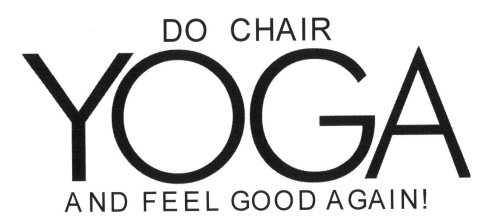

DO CHAIR YOGA AND FEEL GOOD AGAIN!

ALL THE
BENEFITS
WITHOUT
THE FLOOR

BETHANY KNIGHT

Do Chair Yoga and Feel Good Again!
All the Benefits, Without the Floor

Copyright © 2016 Bethany Knight
Second edition September 2017

The information contained herein may not be published, broadcast, rewritten or otherwise distributed without the prior written authority from the author. The information contained herein is presented for educational purposes only, and should not be considered as medical advice. It is supplied so that you can make an informed decision.

ISBN: 978-1519786258

Printed in the United States of America

For more information and how to reach the author, go to:

WWW.YOGABYKNIGHT.COM

Acknowledgments

As Yoga is one of my greatest loves, the gratitude expressed here is fervent. I thank…

*Mother India; Swamis Sivananda, Vishnudevananda, Vivekananda, Rama and Jnaneswariananda, as well as my teacher-trainer Pralad for bringing Yoga to the Western world.

*Vermont Yoga students who taught me how to teach: the faithful Tuesday night Yogis in Glover, the Yogals of Greensboro, and the original Chair Yogis of Riverside Life Enrichment Center in Lyndonville, Craftsbury Community Care Center and Glover Riverside Apartments. Yoga students in Connecticut, especially the Holyogis of Holy Advent Episcopal Church, the Madision Senior Center and Donna Lanzetti's salon.

*Dr. Nedungadi V. Haridas of Chennai; YogaSir of Jhansi and Vipassana Meditation Centers worldwide. Gratitude and affection to the young yogis in the classrooms and orphanages of India, and to the late Boona Rao, a dedicated chair yogi.

*Barbara Monti of Monti and Associates, for inviting me to teach Florida CEOs chair yoga.

*Special appreciation and love to Sujatama, for a home while I wrote this book; to fellow chair Yoga teacher Myrna Lowry Macdonald and other Sivananda practitioners; and to Morgan, my first cyberguide.

*Friend and illustrator Kristin Urie for capturing the simplicity and universality of Yoga in her clean, sweet drawings herein. I joyfully thank her for so perfectly furthering the message. And Sampsa Markkula, for creating the Finnish translation of this book, Jooga, Tie Terveempaan Elamaan (Yoga—the Road to a Healthier Life—Yoga Sitting.)

*My precious family, much metta, for understanding all the winters spent in India. I am a better person because of India and Yoga. Lastly, to those unnamed angels and strangers who've enriched my Yoga journey, bless you all.

*And to Marjorie, for her magic editing eyes!

—Bethany—Yogi Knight

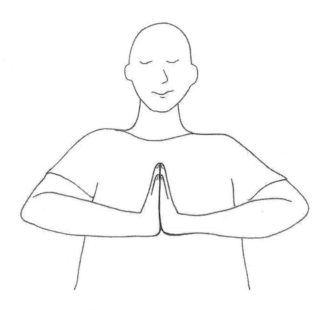

Namaste

TABLE OF CONTENTS

Acknowledgements	3
Welcome to Yoga	6
CHAPTER 1 Your Body, Your Best Friend	11
CHAPTER 2 As the Mind Goes, So Goes the Body	22
CHAPTER 3 Health is Wealth, Yoga Is the Way	31
CHAPTER 4 Your Breath, Your Natural Tranquilizer	36
CHAPTER 5 Yoga Breathing Exercises a.k.a. Pranayama	42
CHAPTER 6 Meditation: Slow Down, Live Long	54
CHAPTER 7 Digging Our Grave with Our Teeth	67
CHAPTER 8 Constipation: Leave It Behind You	72
CHAPTER 9 Chair Yoga for Common Ailments	94
Alphabetical Listing of Common Ailments and Yoga Response	113
Bibliography	177
Glossary	180

WELCOME TO YOGA

*Not in the imagined future
Nor in the remembered past
But only here and only now
Will you find a peace that lasts.*

Anthony was closer to 30 than 40 and a self-made millionaire. He hustled up at the end of a Chair Yoga for CEOs workshop. —Geez, I wish my wife had been here. She can only fall asleep with the TV on, every night, and I'm talking loud. It is making me nuts; now I can't sleep. I don't want her to use drugs, but what can we do?‖ Irving's eyes were full of fatigue, frustration and love.

Anita was stuffing herself at meals and snacking in between, driven by a mindless anxiety she couldn't quiet. Her tension prevented deep, relaxing breaths. Anti-anxiety medications made her tired, but getting fatter and fatter, she felt she had no choice. —I need a way to calm down and focus, to be more disciplined,‖ she said. —I wish I could do Yoga, but I can't get up and down off the floor.‖

Vijay's 75 year old neck was so stiff, he couldn't tip his head back to drink from a bottle. His doctor prescribed pain killers, but there was no magic pill to lubricate the rusty neck. —I can't turn my head when I drive,‖ Vijay worried. —I heard Yoga would be good for me, but I'm afraid to try to get on the floor.‖

Joan was the CEO of a giant accounting business. Managing clients and staff made her feel like a flight controller. —I don't have time for a proper lunch, let alone an hour to exercise every day. Is there something I can do at my desk?‖

Anthony's wife, Anita, Vijay and Joan speak and squeak for millions of sleepless, overworked and anxious people seeking peace, quiet and relief from pain and stiffness. Unable to practice traditional Yoga on the floor because of time, disability, illness or age, they either ignore their needs or opt for extreme measures.

Happily, these four began practicing the poses, breathing and meditation techniques of Chair Yoga, and discovered what you will: from migraines, to indigestion, to depression, Chair Yoga is the answer.

Teaching children, elders, wheelchair users, Alzheimer's patients, businessmen and women, mothers, maximum security prisoners, families, Girl Scouts, preschoolers and college students convinced me anyone can do Yoga and benefit. I am further convinced that no one should miss out on Yoga because s/he can't get down on or up from the floor.

My Sivananda Yoga Teacher's diploma calls for me to —propagate Yoga,‖ and I believe I remain true to the principles when teaching people seated in chairs. Thanks to my first seated and willing students, many confined to a wheelchair or dependent on a walker, I learned that Chair Yoga is lots of fun, too.

CHAIR YOGA FOR WHAT AILS US MENTALLY

What the world needs now, as researchers in Finland define it, is a Culture of Slowness. Without this conscious change in our daily living, neurophysiologists warn that we best prepare for earlier and more common cases of Alzheimer's disease, due to over-stimulation of the cortex.

Little sleep and even less space and time for recovery burns out the frontal cortex. Hundreds of millions of sleep prescriptions are filled monthly around the globe, with many more millions of people self medicating with alcohol and illegal drugs. Antidepressants and anti-anxiety medications have found their way into virtually every family that can afford them.

Our brain and nervous system are paying the price for this addiction to technology. Seated and listening or staring hours a day without bending, stretching or flexing, we shorten arm and leg muscles, freeze up shoulders, wrists, hips and ankles, weaken the spine and slow the bowels.

Spending so little time being still, quiet or alone, we are rapidly aging our brains, damaging our ear drums and living with an extremely challenging level of tension. The connection between stress and health has been long established in medical textbooks; the time has come for families to become conscious of this truth, as record numbers of children are being labeled autistic, learning disabled, bipolar or with attention deficit disorder.

Mom and Dad are busy working 40, 50, 60 hours or more a week, at two or three or four jobs, to earn enough money to run their household. Sitting at home in front of the television, children hear commercials telling them they need something that costs money. (In the US, advertising consumes more than one third of all on-the-air time.) Parents work to exhaustion, so everyone in the family can be alone with his or her cell phone, computer, CD player, ipod and laptop.

When my son was 4 years old, he ran into the kitchen on a Saturday morning, breathless. —Mom, Mom, you gotta buy Cocoa Puffs!‖

—Why?‖ I asked. He knew we didn't buy sugary cereal.

—Because the man on TV said, —Kids, tell your Mom to buy Cocoa Puffs.‖ Many kids do tell their mothers. Marching to the sugar drumbeat and swallowing enormous quantities of manmade foods, children have entered the adult world of obesity.

CHAIR YOGA FOR WHAT AILS US PHYSICALLY

Outliving our joints has become an acceptable, normal occurrence. Most gatherings of people over the age of 55 include at least one ceramic or stainless steel knee and hip. Treating our bodies like automobiles, millions go under the knife, replacing parts and risking infections, even death.

Poor balance causes trips and falls, launching more of us into the surgeon's gloved hands. Our sedentary lifestyle and shallow breathing cause lymph full of waste and toxins to pool in the body, causing illness and disease.

We need a prescription for well being; one that directs us to slow down, stay grateful and in the present. We need to appreciate silence, look within ourselves rather than around the shops for happiness, and to move our bodies as they were intended.

Chair Yoga. Yup. Chair Yoga is what the world needs.

Haughty Americans with just four centuries of history can be quick to discount the powers of Yoga, practiced in the East for more than 50 centuries. That's rather like the Twinkie challenging the banana, don't you think?

Why do we dismiss ancient wisdom, proven over multiple generations to heal, invigorate, restore and maintain physical and mental health and well being?

Because the Man on TV didn't tell us to buy it. Because we don't believe it will be easy enough or instant enough. We are Americans, and not only do we want, we want it now, whether it is instant messaging or all fruits in all seasons of the year. When most of the produce section at the grocery store has flown farther than our grandparents ever did, it is time to stop and think about excess.

Studies show computer users abandon downloads that take longer than 20 seconds. Ketchup bottles are designed to sit upside down, because we can't wait for the goods to flow. News is broadcast as it happens, making evening newspapers obsolete. A Yoga student told me her husband put televisions in every room of the house, including the bathrooms, all broadcasting Fox News 24/7.

On the other side of the world, I was shocked to discover so many Indians are also ignoring their culture's ancient yogic teachings.

Getting to work or school in an Indian city is a form of exercise itself, an exercise in patience, perseverance and creativity. Workdays are easily extended another two or three hours due to transportation. Who has time for Yoga? World _round, it seems making time for ourselves is one of the greatest challenges facing families today.

Living in the instant message age, investing in anything that takes time to bear fruit has little appeal. News is broadcast as it happens, making evening newspapers obsolete.

During my childhood in the 1960s, a family friend gave us a small-framed quotation by Lewis Mumford, to hang in our new, second bathroom. —Today, the degradation of the inner life is symbolized by the fact that the only place sacred from intrusion is the private toilet." With cell phones routinely falling out of pockets and into toilets, poor Mr. Mumford is no longer correct.

CHAIR YOGA FOR WHAT AILS US SPIRITUALLY

When Janet's husband of more than 12 years confessed he had been having an affair for the past three, she lost her bearings, collapsing in tears. Through Chair Yoga, she learned to meditate and found the comfort and hope she desperately needed to continue being a good mother, employee and functioning human being. As a chair Yogi, Janet's recovered her equilibrium and peace of mind. She didn't stay stuck in pain, anger or fear.

Closing each Yoga class, YogaSir, a master teacher in northern India says, —Go out and be kind. Utter no words that will hurt. You can do great things being kind."

Expressing kind words is a good way to start the day. Accessing our inner sense of peace and well being, kindness is also accessible. We can avoid boiling over when stuck in traffic, consuming excessive food and drink and yelling at our families.

Chair Yoga transforms overeating, overspending, chronic pain, persistent sinus problems, backaches, sore feet and mood swings. We become more flexible in our bodies and our thinking. We live longer, healthier lives.

Remain in your seats, please. Welcome to Chair Yoga. You are about to balance and heal yourself, your family and the world.

> *IMPORTANT NOTICE: Never substitute anything written in this book for your own sound judgment about what is best for your body and health. Always consult your physician for medical advice. The stories and the suggested responses to common ailments shared in this book are offered for illustrative purposes only, not prescriptive in any way. I am not a doctor practicing medicine. I am a yogi, practicing Yoga. The names and details used in examples herein are gently altered, to honor individuals' privacy.*

CHAPTER 1

YOUR BODY, YOUR BEST FRIEND

Through Yoga, you may discover that you have more strength and energy than you realized.

Margaret D. Pierce

Yoga is about having a new relationship with your body. Without Yoga or some other fitness program, you may likely harbor great disappointment, if not outright anger and hatred toward your body.

Up until age 40, it was easy for me to alphabetically, chronologically and anatomically recite all of my body's flaws and defects. Fairly superficial when accessing my health as a young woman, my list didn't include legitimate problems, such as a chronic ear infection or an ankle that frequently dislocated. No, my Rotten Roster was a regurgitation of my culture's teachings on how my feminine assets fell short. Not being a Barbie doll, I was a failure, riddled with limitations and self-assessed deformities. How well I remember the dysfunctional relationship I had with my body.

One of the unexpected benefits of moving out of the city into the country was that I no longer could walk in a downtown lined with full-length picture windows. My life-long hobby of judgmentally studying my profile ended! These negative guilt trips generally left me discouraged and full of self-loathing…my hips were too big, my belly not flat enough, my nostrils flared.

A dabbler in Yoga since age 18, when I won a trip to India and took my first Yoga class in Indore, MP, from a real yogi, I was slow in making a serious commitment to its practice.

My fourth decade made Yoga more important, and I began doing some poses daily. My husband was also interested, and we hired a teacher for weekly private lessons.

Without much fanfare, one day our bodies had announced that, indeed, we are aging and possibly, getting arthritic or sick. Aching joints were becoming common, at least while we are awake!

Once committed to Yoga, almost instantly, I began to relate to my body differently. When trying a pose, I was often pleasantly surprised at how comfortably I assumed the position, and how good it felt. My body was not the enemy.

Moving and stretching and bending and balancing and strengthening and breathing were fun. I was happy looking forward to the class, during the class and after the class.

My sense of my body changed. I began to see its strengths, its purpose and its faithfulness. Pose by pose, I became aware of my body as my beautiful vehicle, my lifelong companion on this earthly journey.

THE HONEYMOON

Once we fall in love with our bodies, the honeymoon begins. Because love means we are paying attention, we are listening and respecting, we seek comfort in our own skin.

With this newfound awareness, I started to see connections between the black and blue marks on my legs and hips, and mindlessly crashing through my environment. My ankle stopped twisting and going out underneath me when I noticed the terrain I was traveling. My itchy ear seemed to be tied to putting my head underwater and eating too many sweets.

Wow! My body made sense; it had a story to tell and lessons to teach.

The black and blue marks disappeared, and after a lifetime of such polka dots, it was odd to see bruise-free skin. As a child, I was called Banana Legs, with so many dark spots covering my legs. My husband stopped seeing what he imagined was another man's thumbprint on my thigh!

Through Yoga, we become mindful of our actions. The disappearance of bumps and bruises, caused by carelessness, are among the many changes we experience. YogaSir teaches that

Yoga also helps us avoid accidents, as we become more thoughtful and aware when entering new environments.

Approaching swimming as a sacred act, we regard the water and the moment as Divine. YogaSir instructs, —Touch the water and then your chest and forehead. Place one foot in the water and then the other. Slowly walk around and check out the bottom of the pool or body of water for depth and dangerous objects. Completing this ritual, you are ready to enjoy a safe swim.‖

Becoming a yogi and entering a friendship with your body, persistent ailments and afflictions begin to heal.

As my Yoga practice developed, my need to overeat and overreact diminished. I could sit still for more than five minutes. I stopped picking at my toes, anxiously tearing skin and nails off till they were bleeding or nearly so. I realized fear and anxiety had been propelling me since my early teens, nestled snugly in my gut. I embarked on a campaign to release anxiety for good, and I did.

Yoga has made me a more relaxed, healthy, youthful, patient person. Regardless of your current relationship with your body, its real or perceived limitations or the horsepower of your fear/anxiety engine, Yoga will transform you, too.

Chronic physical problems are ideally addressed by Yoga. Rather than another prescription for your migraines or sinus congestion, why not try Yoga? Neck aches disappear, constipation vanishes, and throats get clear.

Yoga is about getting to know yourself and how your body functions, seeing abnormalities differently.

Not an instant cure, quick fix or one time procedure, Yoga is a new way of life, a way of being with yourself and others. And with Chair Yoga, you needn't say, —I can't get on the floor, so I can't do Yoga.‖ After years of working with senior citizens and their caregivers in a variety of settings, I'm convinced Yoga benefits anyone committed to learn.

OUR BODY IS OUR BEST FRIEND

Learning to listen to and interpret the signs and symptoms the body sends is both fascinating and fulfilling. From a Yoga standpoint, poor digestion or a dreadful headache are no longer handled by a mindless trip to the pharmacy so you can gulp down pills.

Awakened to your body's deep interest in your well-being, you see discomfort and disease as the flashing light on the dashboard, directing you to ―check engine‖. Aches and painful sensations are no longer random or met with impatience and prescriptions. Rather, we thank our body for getting our attention, calling for more self-observation.

To assist you in your own self-discovery about a nagging health problem, take the Six Question Quiz. Use it to work through a specific chronic health or physical problem, such as persistent backaches or indigestion.

Six Question Quiz

1. What is your history with this problem? Sit quietly and recall your earliest memory or awareness of its presence. (―I was 16, in French class, feeling a lot of stress about studying, and I got my first blinding migraine.‖) Look closely at what triggers or worsens your condition (―When my parents stay for a few days, my psoriasis flares up.‖) Search for warning signs that occur prior to a full-blown problem (―I know I am going to get sick when I feel so utterly exhausted, so completely beat, I just want to sleep.‖) Review and list all the treatments you have tried to cure yourself of this problem.

2. What is your own theory about why you have this problem? The body's default state is wellness, so why are you suffering? Could infirmity be serving you in some way? What could be the pay off for you, what makes the problem repeat? (―I hate to say no when a friend asks me to come to her grandson's engagement party. But when my arthritis is acting up, I have no choice, I tell them if I could, I would, but I can't.‖) Who are you responsible for? That is, who

counts on you for significant support? Children? Spouse? Parents? Employees? Pets? Others?

3. What do you do to relax? Ingesting or consuming tranquilizing substances does not count. Nor does doing something you also do for work, such as computer activity or house cleaning. Ideally, true relaxation involves no technology or medication. How much true relaxation do you program into your week?

4. In question 2 you identified the pay off or value of your problem, how it actually functions as a backhanded or backdoor way of helping you. Now, for some more soul searching: what is the cost of this problem? What is it costing you to suffer and not be healed? What are you missing? (―I can't go to my son's soccer games because I can't walk that far.‖) Honestly examine just what price you are paying for ignoring your well-being. What is this costing your loved ones? (―My daughter cried because I am too fat to take a dance class with her.‖)

5. How much do you truly want to change? How much are you willing to make the changes required? Can you imagine finding a new, healthier way to achieve what your problem currently does for you? Reread your answer to question 2. Are you ready to be honest in your life, and speak your truth, or will you continue to have your body be your spokesperson?

Once you decide you are worth it and healing is your goal, it is time to turn to Chair Yoga for the way.

Like a difficult person in our lives, physical problems and illness are our teachers. Incidents that cause us to examine our lives and make changes are our *Monica Lewinsky Moment* (apologies to Monica.) Remember her, the young White House intern who became involved with then U.S. President Bill Clinton?

Early in their marriage, Bill and wife Hillary became aware of his dangerous sexual addiction. Opportunities to deal with the problem arose regularly. But like most of us, busy, preoccupied and avoiding conflict at all costs, the Clintons managed to squint and overlook Bill's dysfunction.

We can all relate to this finely tuned capacity to avoid the obvious. Massage clients routinely come to me in great pain: a frozen shoulder, a cramped hand, a debilitating backache. ―How long has this been going on?‖ I ask.

The answer comes in years, not days or weeks or months.

Years! Waiting years to get help, to seek relief? ―What have you done for it?‖ I ask.

―Ignore it!‖ and ―Hate it!‖ are the two most common answers.

Like Bill and Hillary, we hope denial works. Of course, the joke is on us, because denial only works until we receive such a giant wake up call, that closing our eyes or crying ―conspiracy‖ doesn't work. Our *Monica Lewinsky Moment* has arrived, the incident or event that stops us in our tracks, blows the whistle and announces, ―I demand your attention.‖

When *Monica* manifests as a physical problem, appears as a stroke, emergency surgery, a terrible fall, an autoimmune syndrome. Shaken awake by circumstances we can no longer handle by ignoring and hating, we are often stunned by the bad news.

―I have diabetes! I can't believe it!‖ we cry, pretending the diagnosis is a total shock, from out of the blue.

Are we so disconnected from our bodies, that we never considered the consequences of overeating? Do we think eating heavy, high calorie meals late at night is good self care?

The good news is Yoga reverses many dire conditions. If you are like that old soft cucumber at the market and at least 50 percent intact, Yoga will help. And for those cucumbers too soft to be sold, Yoga will make you more comfortable and teach you to no longer fear illness and death.

FINDING YOUR SILVER LINING

Our bodies are perfectly designed. We are given multiple chances to heal and recover fully from a range of maladies. Of course, healing is easiest when we pay careful attention the first time we notice the ―check engine‖ light is flashing. But if you're like my friend who stuck a post-it note over that dash feature, your healing requires greater effort.

Okay, so something is off, you don't feel like yourself. You've had loose bowel movements for a week. Or worse, no movements at all. Maybe you have a bitter taste in your mouth and notice white scum on your tongue.

Once you adopt a Yoga way of living, you enter into a new relationship with your body, recognizing it isn't the enemy you must hate and ignore. Rather, you seek to care for it, asking —Why did you get my attention this way? What are you trying to tell me?‖

My friend Dolly can never say no to her children or grandchildren. With dozens of them, she is forever being asked to baby-sit, transport, cook, make birthday cake, shop for Halloween costumes, the list is endless. A loving woman, Dolly loves to be loved and needed, but she can't maintain the pace her family demands. Unable to say —no‖ to anyone, Dolly lets her body do the talking: she ends up in bed for weeks with mysterious symptoms, often being rushed to the hospital by ambulance. Dolly lets her body somatize what she doesn't verbalize. The payoff is she can get out of saying —no‖ and still gets rest. The cost is obvious, wearing herself out, destroying her immunity, missing out on the fun.

—We know, even if our surgeons and internists don't, that we are connected with our bodies,‖ writes Dr. Ronald J. Glasser. —The catch in our breath when we are startled, the tension in our guts when we're worried, the exhaustion we feel from our anxiety, are as much a part of our illness as are the bacteria, viruses and auto-antibodies which attack us, and can in fact be just as debilitating and just as deadly.‖

DON'T DOUBT YOUR INTUITION, YOUR INSTINCTS

As always, it is easier to see the lessons others need to learn. But what about you? What is the payoff and cost of your infirmities?

When you begin a dialogue with your body, don't doubt your intuition or your instincts. It is important to listen to the thoughts that pop into your head.

BEING WOMEN AND MEN OF FAITH AND PRACTICING YOGA, WE CAN HEAL THE WORLD

More than a few of my fellow Christians have timidly entered a Yoga class, worried that somehow this healing practice could put them at cross purposes with the Cross.

My answer is that, for me, Yoga has deepened my spiritual life and made me more open and receptive to the Scriptures. By stilling my mind, and learning how to be more mindful and present, I am a more loving person, of others and myself. Jesus taught us to, —Love one another as you love yourself.‖ With Yoga, I have found a way to do just that.

A Protestant minister once banned me from teaching Yoga in his Vermont church. His reason?

—When you still the mind,‖ he told me, —You let the devil in.‖ I smiled and said, —Well, maybe your mind, but not mine. I've never experienced anything but relief when I am quiet.‖

Yoga is a form of self-care, not a selfish avocation. When we take care of ourselves, we honor this temple of flesh and everyone in our life benefits.

Imagine an old rain barrel in the yard, filling with water gradually, storm by storm. Now, imagine the drops of rain are people and the barrel is the continent you live on. As more people begin to practice Yoga and meditation, your continent fills with more harmony, peace and wellness.

Once enough people embrace a healthy way of life, the barrel full of drops of water will overflow; beyond your family, neighborhood, state, country and continent, flooding the whole world with the good news of joyful living.

Your decision to practice Yoga could be the drop that pushes the water over the edge of the barrel, watering parched people everywhere with truth and love. And you thought making time for Yoga was selfish!

Yoga classes are open to students of all faith traditions, as well as those who subscribe to no particularly belief system. I have taught Christians, Hindus, Sikhs, Jews, Jains, Buddhists, Muslims, Humanists, agnostics, atheists and more. Somehow, in our diversity, we all are drawn to practice Yoga and reap the benefits. Our classes are a microcosm of the world, how the globe could live cooperatively.

How you arrive at and participate in a Yoga class is precisely how you function in your life.

Do you come prepared, healthy, happy, hopeful? Are you ready to learn and be flexible and experience blessings? Do you believe you can handle the moment?

Are you dressed comfortably? Do you have what you need to create good conditions? Do you feel ready to laugh and play?

Do you enjoy the presence of others? How do you relate to them? As competitors? Potential problems? Different? Greater? Lesser? Friends? Do you allow yourself to receive the blessings of the class? Of the day?

The Universe is always seeking balance; we automatically feel glad when needed rain or sun come. This same desire for balance, or homeostasis, is within each one of us. As we seek and find our balance, we help tip the Universal Scale to the center.

Why do we believe that a doctor or other health care practitioner who spends 15 or 30 minutes with us will have a better idea about us than we do? Over the years, we have surrendered more and more of our identity and sense of self to others, to the outside, to the external. We need others to tell us we are smart and attractive. We look to designers and manufacturers to tell us what to wear. Thanks to marketers, we long ago forgot we are masters of our own destiny, and that there is a treasure chest inside, full of ideas, answers and wisdom.

Answering the **Six Question Quiz**, we see the body protects us from perceived threats and derives a benefit or payoff by allowing poor health. Our challenge is to listen to ourselves before sickness takes hold.

When we don't speak up, our bodies do. Stated even more directly, if you don't say no, your body will. Sickness is the Universe's way of getting your attention, throwing you on your back or down on your knees to be more honest in your life. Being honest means your life becomes easier.

Rather than dive into fear mode when you need healing, remember everything that happens to you is for your highest good. Time and again, clients I work with who willingly find the lessons and the meaning of their setback, come out of it stronger, happier and more authentic. All life experience is purposeful.

The truth is we aren't two separate entities, a separate mind and separate body. Yoga teaches us that the mind is throughout the body, in every cell, not just housed in the brain. To confirm this truth in your own life, recall a moment when an unpleasant thought came to mind and you felt your stomach tighten up, or a sharp pain in the belly.

That said; don't jump to the tempting conclusion that you consciously cause illness. We are not conscious of any such activity on this level. We aren't causing illness, but we do allow it. We permit the conditions to arise that host illness because, until we wake up to this pattern, our body uses it to prevent more pain, more assaults on our well-being. Awakened to the pattern, we find a powerful motivation to heal, to be free.

For your body, healing and freedom is the same thing. When I became a Catholic, I had trouble remembering what to say prior to receiving the communion bread and wine. For the first few Sundays, I would say, —Lord, I am not worthy to receive you, but only say the word, and I shall be free.‖

One Sunday, sitting next to a friend with good diction, I finally and clearly heard, —Lord, I am not worthy to receive you, but only say the word and I shall be healed.‖

Free. Healed. For me, they were the same thing. Free of pain. Healed of pain.

Chapter 2

As the Mind Goes, So Goes the Body

What you think you become.
The Buddha

We all love to read newspaper stories of true heroics: a man lifts a car and frees a trapped child, a stranger enters a burning building and rescues a young mother. While such efforts defy our rational thinking, we know they are possible

Extraordinary incidents dramatically prove the power of the mind over the body. Accepting the mind's ability to cause super human feats, it is an easy leap to recognize the incredible power our thoughts wield when it comes to our health.

In our own lives, on a small scale, we see the influence of mind on body all the time. Ever wake with a sore throat or headache, on a day you dreaded a meeting or responsibility? How many times have you felt rotten, perhaps limping around the house with a sore foot, when someone walks in whom you don't want to trouble with your pain? You begin to walk normally. Or a friend unexpectedly drops over and invites you out for a movie… and you cheerfully walk out of the house without a limp?

What about those first days on a new job, when you had inexplicable diarrhea? I remember my first two weeks as a reporter at the Adrian Daily Telegram, in Adrian, Michigan. My bowels poured like a garden hose. Did I have some serious disease? Was this a sign of cancer?

At the doctor's office, my physician listened, examined me and told me a story. —When I was playing high school football, before every game I would go out behind the stadium and throw up. Then, I was ready to play.‖ He suggested I come back in two weeks if the loose movements hadn't cleared up by then. Of course, normal bowels returned soon after the appointment.

Once we willingly embrace the intimate connection between our thinking and our health, we discover how much sway we have over our well being.

Harvard researchers published findings from a study that explored the link between hostility and lung function. Even at the beginning of the study, men with the highest anger ratings had the poorest lung function, and their condition deteriorated over the period of the study.

According to one of the study's authors, Dr. Paul Lehrer, —Stress-related factors are known to depress immune function and increase susceptibility to, or exacerbate a host of diseases and disorders. Indeed, it is hard to find a disease for which emotion or stress plays absolutely no part in symptom severity, frequency, or intensity of flare-ups.‖

Other studies have discovered that thoughts of hopelessness or helplessness can lead to anxiety and depression. Negative thoughts were once considered symptoms of anxiety and depression, but brilliant scientists like Abraham Low, Aaron Beck and Albert Ellis found that specific types of thinking actually cause mood disorders. Alter the way you think and nervous system problems disappear.

Perhaps no group has been more starved for the gift of Chair Yoga than returning veterans of conflict. Hundreds of thousands of veterans return to the US with permanent, life altering injuries. Traumatic brain injury, severe depression, blindness and the multiple loss of limbs has become common. Our excellent first responders in the battlefield are able to save soldiers whose wounds would have resulted in certain death in earlier wars.

But getting back to anything that resembles a normal life is sometimes overwhelming, and directly related to the rising rate of suicides among the military.

The Give Back Yoga Foundation (www.givebackYoga.org) offers free Yoga and meditation resources to veterans across the US. One of the program's many success stories is a Viet Nam vet named Paul, who had struggled with post traumatic stress disorder, PTSD, for 40 years. —When I was told I was going to do Yoga,‖ Paul recalled, —I thought of rolling around the floor in a leotard.‖ Now a true believer, Paul considers Yoga, —the most useful survival skill I know.‖

CREATING CANCER TO RETIRE EARLY

One of my first clients in India was a lovely woman in the last stages of uterine cancer. Invited by her sister to do some healing work, I visited with Usha and listened to her life story. A wife and mother, she had aspired to a career in banking. But promotion after promotion evaded her; with far less experienced men receiving advancements and postings she sought.

Early on, she began to realize the bank was not where she wanted to work, but a combination of anger and stubbornness kept her from quitting. —I was determined to get somewhere, no matter how much they ignored me,‖ she said, her eyes burning with pain.

When a supervisor hinted that Usha's willingness to accept an unpopular assignment in a faraway hill station would result in a desired promotion, she agreed and moved. —My daughter and husband were angry I left them, but I felt I had no choice,‖ she recalled.

Completing her tour in the outback, Usha was again denied a more prestigious position. At that point, she confronted management with her frustration. —They told me I could always quit if I wasn't happy,‖ she said. —But by then I had invested in the retirement plan. I asked if I could take my retirement with me and go.‖

Bank policy dictated no early withdrawal of retirement funds, except, Usha said, —They joked that if I got cancer, I could retire early.‖

Listening to her own voice state this fact, Usha became silent. —I got cancer,‖ she said to herself and me.

In our time together, Usha did some beautiful healing work. She got in touch with her heart's desire, a long held secret wish to teach art to the poorest of India's poor, the rag pickers' children. An artist who long ago had stopped making art, she yearned to create with children. We discussed the fact that cancer appeared in her uterus, the organ of creation. —No accident,‖ we concluded, as she had ignored her own yearnings to create art and teach.

Nutritionist and healer Hanna Kroeger wrote, —If we have happy and constructive thoughts, energy will follow these kinds of thoughts and build a healthy environment and healthy body....If you are slowed down, frustrated in reaching your goal and unable to express yourself creatively, you become ill. Creative expression is the most important factor in staying well.‖

After so much surgery, radiation and chemotherapy, Usha was very sick and weak. She made the decision to leave this earth. Her husband and daughter were not visiting. She decided that she could find the most peace by praying daily for the rag pickers' children, since she was too tired to do more. Her death, with her devoted sister at her bedside, was peaceful.

Wakening up to the mind body connection before we are terminally ill is certainly a preferred way to live!

DON'T MOVE SO YOU CAN'T MOVE

When I met Diane, she was in her sixth year of suffering from an unidentified type of palsy. Doctors were baffled by her condition, and without any other ideas, treated her for a neuromuscular disorder. She was taking 14 pills daily for tremors and periodic freezing of her limbs and neck. Once a gregarious, happy teacher, this wife and mother was confined to the home by the disability.

Listening to Diane's story, I heard about a husband who moved the family at least once a year, if not more often. Relocating so frequently, the couple could never buy or establish a home. Diane came to hate this regular uprooting. But, unable to tell her husband she didn't want to move, her body did it for her.

—I just can't move! I'm stuck! And in between my son and my husband, I am stuck in the middle.‖

Playing back her own words to her, I asked Diane what she thought was going on. —Oh, my God,‖ she said, wide-eyed, —I didn't tell him the truth, because I didn't want to upset him. But I am sick and tired of moving, and I want him to spend some time with our son.‖

Sick and tired of moving! The moment Diane recognized the truth of her condition, she began to see the connection between her thinking and her symptoms. When she could mentally relax, she noticed a loose and flexible neck, and continued to watch her body let go and stop doing the talking for her. She sat with her husband and told him the truth, staying in their apartment as he left for yet another job in another city.

In case after case, we can see the mind's powerful role in dictating our health. *Chapter 8 identifies the thinking that impairs healthy bowel action.* Virtually every bodily function is susceptible to our mind's persuasion. Check the bibliography for further reading, particularly the work of Louise Hay and Dr. Gabor Mate, on this subject.

Hay, a California metaphysical healer, writes, —The body is a mirror of our inner thoughts and beliefs. The body is always talking to us, if we will only take the time to listen. Every cell within your body responds to every single thought you think and every word you speak.‖

Mate, a Vancouver physician, writes, —Physiological stress is the link between personality traits and disease. Certain traits, otherwise known as coping styles, magnify the risk for illness by creating the likelihood of chronic stress. Common to them all is a diminished capacity for emotional communication.‖

Our bodies clearly listen to our thinking and our speaking. If we are afraid and don't say what we need to say, if we have words caught in our throats, there's a good chance we'll develop a cough or some other problem, as our body works to dislodge our truth.

THE BODY WON'T PRETEND

Working with a church organist who developed a tic in her eye, we approached her condition like detectives. —What happened just prior to the tic's arrival?‖

Maria described a luncheon she had attended with the pastor of the church. New to his job, he asked to meet with her, expressing a desire to get acquainted. —But after 30 minutes of listening to him talk about himself, I began to wonder if he really wanted to know me,‖ Maria said.

—Finally he said, ‗Well, I think we should get down to the real reason we got together,'‖ she recalled. —I opened my mouth to tell him about my love of the organ and how I started to play it when he interrupted, ‚I want to approve all the music you teach the choir and chose to be sung at services.'‖

Stunned by the pastor's request, Maria said she felt very angry and hurt.

I asked if she let him know her feelings.

—No. I was a lady,‖ she replied.

—A lady with a tic,‖ I laughed, pointing out that her body wasn't as willing to appear undisturbed by his ambush. —You were blindsided, Maria. What happens when someone comes at you with their fist?‖

She blinked. The tic disappeared. We saw how her body had done its best to defend her from a perceived attack.

If we are willing to honestly and openly look at our lives and our health, each of us can find similar stories of illness, injury or pain that actually can be translated into concrete messages about our life circumstances.

The fun begins when we decide to get ahead of the game, and learn to direct our thinking before the mind allows disease or infirmity to take up residence. Yoga is about training the mind and the body.

Can the mind be trained or retrained to —Just Say No?‖

One of the most famous answers to this question appears in the book, <u>Alone</u>, the story of Admiral Byrd's 1934 trip to the South Pole. His mission appeared to be ending in failure, and he decided he was going to die alone in his tent. He wrote a note to those who would find him and lay down to die.

Byrd had an unexpected sensory memory from his childhood came to mind that fateful night. His body recalled another time he felt resignation and defeat, while a student at the Naval Academy. In pain at the end of championship wrestling match, his body experienced this same urge to give up.

But at that moment, he realized he didn't want to disappoint his mother, who was sitting in the stands. With the power of a determined thought, Byrd persevered and won the match.

This time in the bleak and barren Antarctic wasteland, he wondered if he could listen to his body and direct his mind to again persevere. He could and he did.

The belief or sense that we are worth standing up for, that life is worth living, is one of the most powerful tools a human being can use.

Psychotherapist Lawrence LeShan has spent more than 30 years working with chronically ill patients, and along the way discovered the connection between wellness and the heart's desire. Again, he links the body with the mind, seeing how immunity can be boosted with joy.

Rather than only treating problems the patient presents, Dr. LeShan also focuses on what they are looking forward to, what they are enthusiastic about. By discovering what a patient longs to do and encouraging him or her to chase dreams, Dr. LeShan helps patients become strong and recover from a myriad of auto immune diseases.

One patient presented at his office with a terminal cancer tumor. She had basically accepted her diagnosis, and expressed no real interest in getting well. Dr. LeShan spent time with her, looking for that spark that would cause her to choose wellness.

After several sessions together, she shared a childhood dream to play the piano. Arranging for lessons and learning to play the piano, this wife and mother's tumor shrank and she lived a long life, playing her piano daily.

YOGA FOR YOUR MIND AND BODY

Students of Yoga are not surprised by these stories of mind and body communication and connection. For the yogi, the body is not a mystery. Rather, it is an archive, storing information and memories that influence health and well being.

Spending time daily with your body on a mat, physical awareness expands. The aching hip is seen as the consequence of the prior day's long bus ride. The sore arch is tied to wearing those cute but uncomfortable sandals to the party.

Yoga tunes you in to you. Like Admiral Byrd, you can become still and let your body teach you to survive and thrive.

Body Scan

Sit quietly and scan your body. Using your left arm as a meter, stretch it and lift up, inhaling until it is extended over your head, pointing at ceiling. As the arm moves up, scan the entire side of the body, looking for aches and pains, stresses and strains. Notice if you feel any tension, discomfort or awkwardness. Are you carrying any anger, disappointment, fear, worry, emptiness? Inhale the healing energy of *Prana* into those spaces you identify. *See Chapter 5 on Prana, the life force.* As you bring your long, strong arm back down to the side, exhale whatever is no longer serving you, and let it go. Exhale the waste, the old stories. Use your arm as a meter as long as you wish, until your left side feels balanced.

Repeat on your right side.

If painful stories or incidents come up, use your mind and consciously choose not to let these thoughts take root in your body. Picture a barren desert where nothing can grow. See the tumbleweed blowing by. Watch your hurts and pain dry up and pass by.

Slide Show Meditation

Sit comfortably and quietly. Close your eyes. In your mind, set up a slide show. For folks over 50, we remember the old Carousel slide projectors. Our children see a computer screen with images flashing across it!

Project a series of pictures on the screen of a problem you are having with your body. A stiff neck, slipped disk, migraine headache, whatever bothers you, step outside yourself and watch yourself experiencing this challenge. Reverse the slide show and watch what preceded the pain, that is, what occurred prior to you seeing your health compromised. Who were you with? What did they say? What did you feel? What were you doing?

If an accident or injury appears, observe your state of mind at the time of the incident. Were you preoccupied or distracted? What had you been thinking about? Were you neglecting yourself in some way, or ignoring your needs? Is there any anger you need to deal with? Is there a need for forgiveness or apologies?

Continue to hit the forward and reverse arrows of your slide show, getting as much information as you can about your circumstances. Are lessons appearing? Can you see what your body is trying to show you or teach you? Why have you been stopped at this moment? What requires your attention? Stay with these thoughts and pictures as long as you are comfortable.

Second Slide Show

Again, sit comfortably and quietly. Close your eyes. This meditation can follow your first slide show immediately or be done later. The first slide show was about the past, this one is of the present and future, the story that you are about to create.

See yourself in perfect health, with all your ailments healed. See yourself doing the things you have longed to do. Is that you skiing? Hiking? Dancing? Enjoy the pictures, in ballrooms or on mountaintops, in a canoe or on horseback. Where will your good health take you?

Notice who is enjoying this good health with you. Look into their eyes and your own, see the vitality and energy. Celebrate your health and well being.

As you watch this Travelogue of the Future, be conscious of how your body feels. Experience the pleasant, happy feelings throughout your body. Enjoy the lightness of your being. The brain responds to stories and reality the same way, so by visualizing good health and good fun, your brain produces the same chemical responses it would during the actual event.

Enjoy the comfort of these pictures, and accept the fact that you are creating your future, right now, in your mind. See how you can make your thoughts real, how you can manifest your heart's desire. Stay with these thoughts and pictures as long as you are comfortable.

Chapter 3

HEALTH IS WEALTH, YOGA IS THE WAY

*Health is wealth,
peace of mind is happiness
and Yoga shows the way.*

       Swami Vishnudevananda

Swami Vishnudevananda, one of my gurus, taught, —Health is wealth, peace of mind is happiness and Yoga shows the way.‖ How does this work?

Dedicating time in your week or day for Yoga means you consciously choose to remove yourself from the rat race and exhale. You sit in a nice, well-ventilated room and quiet your mind. You take time to breathe and release the tension held in your neck, back, shoulders, chest, feet…wherever your stress storage units are located.

By treating yourself to some simple breathing and stretches, you start a loving relationship with your body and assure yourself sound health and real happiness.

Twinges and hitches in your side no longer go unnoticed. Gradually, your awareness starts to shift from being *Out There* focused to *In Here* focused. You enter a mutual aid agreement with your body, that it will no longer be forgotten or overlooked. You learn which breathing and poses, known as *Pranayama* and *Asanas*, are best suited to your constitution. You become licensed to operate your vehicle, your body.

My fellow Sivananda certified teacher, Canadian Myrna Lowry, gives her students, —a wee talk, on how we can incorporate Yoga into our daily life.

—Yoga anytime, anywhere,‖ she says. —We can do our breathing exercises and meditations while waiting for an appointment; our balances while waiting for supper (or doughnuts) to cook; and the Lion while driving the car (when no one is looking) it could help with road-rage, no?

—In other words we can bring our Yoga practice into our daily lives, making it a part of us and us a part of it – the true union of Yoga. See page 168 to learn the Roaring Lion.

I would add to Myrna's advice that, for yogis, waiting for the microwave is never boring, and TV commercials suddenly have a healthy purpose!

When asked about the power of Yoga, Swami Vishnudevananda wrote:

—Yoga is a life self-discipline based on the tenets of simple living and high thinking. The body is the temple or vehicle for the soul, and has specific requirements, which must be fulfilled for it to function smoothly and supply the optimum mileage. These requirements can be seen metaphorically in relationship to those of another vehicle. An automobile requires five things: a lubricating system, a battery, a cooling system, fuel and a responsible driver behind the wheel.

A disciple of Swami Sivananda, an Indian physician who opened Yoga Forest academies in the 1800s in India, Swami Vishnudevananda is often credited with bringing this 5000 year old tradition to North America. As articulated by Vishnudevananda, the five principles of Sivananda Yoga are:

Proper Exercise (*Asanas*) acts as a lubricating routine for the joints, muscles, ligaments, tendons and other parts of the body, by increasing circulation and flexibility.

Proper Breathing (*Pranayama*) aids the body in connecting to its battery, the solar plexus, where tremendous potential energy is stored. When tapped through *Pranayama*, this energy is released for physical and mental rejuvenation.

Proper Relaxation *(Savasana)* cools down the system, as does the radiator of a car. Relaxation is Nature's way of recharging the body.

Proper Diet *(Vegetarian)* provides the correct fuel for the body. Optimum utilization of food, air, water and sunlight is essential. This is a very personal decision; if you wish to continue eating meat, you can still practice yoga!

Positive Thinking and Meditation puts you in control. The intellect is purified. The lower nature is brought under conscious control through steadiness and concentration of the mind.

The literal meaning of the word Yoga is ―to yoke,‖ from the Sanskrit verb *Yuj*. Chair Yoga provides us with several opportunities for yoking or union.

Disciplining ourselves to do specific breathing and poses, we yoke the body and mind together, using the breath. Harmonizing ourselves with the community at large, we begin to feel more connected or yoked to others and to something larger than ourselves.

For those who are fast living and goal oriented, Yoga is particularly welcome because of its non-competitive nature. Students are not pitted against each other in class, no one is ranked as better or best. Some teachers maintain this single factor is why fewer men practice Yoga, as it cuts against the traditional play-to-win male stereotype. Rather, we pursue our practice from our own starting point, remembering it is called *practice*, not *perfect*. Mastery is a possibility out there for all of us, but it isn't why we do our Yoga. We do our Yoga for this day.

After years of practicing and teaching Yoga without formal credentialing, I decided to seek teacher certification in 2003, through the Sivananda organization.

In 2004, I completed training in Ayurvedic massage, again through Sivananda, again, to receive formal credentialing, again, after years of practice.

In the Hatha Yoga tradition, Sivananda has kept its simple, pure roots in the Indian traditions, resisting the pressures to Westernize or glamorize the teaching. (www.sivananda.org)

One of India's greatest living Yoga masters, Swami Ramdev, dreams of a disease free world, achieved through the mass practice of Ayurvedic remedies and Yoga.

—When we inhale, it is not only the air or oxygen that enters our body, but also the Divine Vital Energy that permeates the entire Universe, which keeps the body alive, Ramdev says. (www.divyaYoga.com). He teaches that these ancient sciences will bring peace and happiness to mankind, end the multibillion-dollar international weapons business and the need for allopathic medicines.

Pure Yoga is done lying, sitting or standing on the floor, but learning the basics sitting in a chair is no less pure. For the serious student, all of the outcomes are the same.

Sometimes, the chair is just an introduction to Yoga and the student ends up buying a mat and surrendering to the floor.

Mari was such a student. Not athletic or physically active, she signed up for a Chair Yoga class and was surprised by how good and relaxed she felt after an hour of practice. One night, she decided to stay after the Chair Yoga class and try Yoga on the floor. I loaned her a mat and Mari was again surprised by how much Yoga she was able to do. For the rest of the Yoga series, she came to both Chair Yoga and Mat Yoga classes.

At different times in our lives, getting up and down from the floor can be an impossible feat. Hip surgery, extreme stiffness due to arthritis or inactivity and being overweight are common reasons Chair Yoga is the best way to practice Yoga.

New Chair Yoga students are forever exclaiming, —I had no idea what a workout I get sitting down! I was sweating! I even got winded!

When Boona heard she could improve her balance doing Chair Yoga, she asked for a private class.

—My granddaughter is getting married, and I want to dance at her wedding, she told me. Inactive and relying on steroid shots for pain, Boona's balance was too risky for floor Yoga.

I taught her two private classes a week for several months while I was living outside of Bangalore, and Boona was an eager student. She graduated to some standing poses, using the back of her chair for support. Her balance and confidence continued to grow stronger, and yes, she danced at the wedding.

When Annie came to a floor Yoga class for the first time, she experienced a lot pain lying on the floor. Suffering from an old tailbone injury and a lack of flexibility, she decided Yoga was not for her.

—Please, Annie, I suggested, —Try Chair Yoga next week. Give it a chance; I think if you bring a pillow to sit on, you will love it.

Laughing and smiling through her first Chair Yoga class, Annie was delighted to find she could practice Yoga actively and pain free. You will be, too.

CHAPTER 4

YOUR BREATH, YOUR NATURAL TRANQUILIZER

*"You literally work at
one fifth of your potential
when you don't get enough oxygen.
Your body slows down, gains weight, and becomes
even more stubborn about changing."*

Pam Grout

The underlying factor in all infections, allergies, hormonal disturbances, nutritional deficiencies, nervous disorders, disease, fatigue, memory problems and other disordered energy is the result of a, ―Bad breathing epidemic,‖ according to Dr. Sheldon Saul Hendler, <u>The Oxygen Breakthrough</u>. As respiration is the power behind all organ and glandular activity, muscle contraction and thought, breath truly is the boss, directing the human experience of life.

Standard laboratory tests often show a large number of patients have irregularly high levels of carbon dioxide in their blood, when all other blood levels are normal. Such abnormal readings confirm that people routinely do not inhale enough oxygen or exhale enough carbon dioxide, resulting in fatigue, muddy thinking and inefficient operation of cells, tissues, muscles and organs.

Inhaling and exhaling 8.7 million times a year, the difference between robust breathing and shallow or futile breathing is literally a matter of life or death. Shallow or futile breathing, inadequate breathing is practiced by almost all of us, which means we pull in only about 20 percent of the oxygen we need to live a robust, vital life. While our lungs can hold nearly 2 gallons of oxygen (opera singers and skiers are among the few who do fill their tanks), we generally operate on a little more than a liter, between 2 and 3 pints. Shallow breathers use only the chest muscles, thus filling only the middle and upper lobes of the lungs. The lungs are incredibly prepared to serve us; with a surface area half the size of a tennis court, we can inhale more than 24 pounds of air a day.

When we inhale, the muscular cone-shaped sheet called the diaphragm, between the lungs and the abdominal cavity, moves downward, pushing everything in the cavity down. During exhalation, the diaphragm moves back up.

Beginning a disciplined program of focused breathing can inspire those who want to start an exercise program. Most personal trainers agree that the greatest benefit of a physical workout is the development of deep, nourishing breathing.

Beyond toning the body, breath bridges the inside and the outside, the known field to the unknown, seen to unseen, the conscious and the unconscious parts of the mind.

American Olympic athletes competing in a variety of sports are now training with breath control under water, learning to stay relaxed and in control of their breathing. By mastering the ability to stay underwater for more than four minutes, the Olympians can then achieve the same sense of calm in stressful competition, such as the top of a ski jump or during an aerial trick on a snowboard.

—Divers enter a kind of meditative state, fill their lungs with air, then close their throat in a way that relaxes the chest wall, Matthew Futterman reported in the Wall Street Journal. Sounds like Pranayama to a Yogi!

Thich Nhat Hanh, the Buddhist monk and author, says there should be a breathing room in every house, a room to go and breathe.

THE FIVE GIFTS OF BREATH

1—Your Idea Maker

- Fuels the brain; no breath, no thought.

- Twenty percent of the oxygen we inhale is sent to the brain, though it accounts for just three percent of your body weight.
- Ancient Greeks used the same word for brain and diaphragm, acknowledging the vital connection between breath and thought.

2—Your Natural Tranquilizer

- Exhale lowers your blood pressure.
- Signals the brain to release our inbuilt feel good drug…endorphins… the same way eating does.
- Is intertwined with emotion. When we're frightened or think a negative thought, our breath speeds up and gets shallow.
- When we are discouraged and overwhelmed, we sigh.
- When we want to avoid crying or laughing or screaming at a time we perceive as inappropriate, we hold the breath.
- When we are amazed, we say life takes our breath away.
- A calm and quiet mind is intimately associated with slow, deep, rhythmic breathing.
- Full deep breaths ramp up our overall immunity and increase our ability to handle stress. Breathing deeply, we get lighter as we let go of disappointment, pain and painful memories stored on a cellular level.
- Women giving birth are always instructed to focus fully on deep, rhythmic breathing, to get through delivery.

When our guts are knotted with anxiety, our calves full of rage and our head pounding with tension, breath provides the fastest fix. Recent studies at Western universities confirm that deep breathing is extremely effective in handling depression, anxiety and stress-related problems.

The sympathetic nervous system is stimulated in times of stress and anxiety, dispensing adrenaline and other specialized hormones. We can easily become cortisol junkies when this system is fired up too often and for too long. A host of health problems arise. When we train ourselves to breathe deeply during tense times, the breath alerts the parasympathetic nervous system to balance mood swings and calm the body.

When sitting through a frustrating meeting at work or eating or with irritating friends or family, don't forget to breathe!

3—Your Metabolism Manager

- Fires up your digestion.
- Causes the diaphragm, if the breath is deep enough, to actually push against the stomach, nudging it into action.
- Stimulates the enzymes that burn fat. Speeds up the metabolism, fuels the burning of glucose and fat. When stressed, the body typically burns glycogen, not fat. But through deep breathing we can trigger the body to relax and switch from sugar to fat burning.
- Stimulates food absorption.
- Burns five calories with each liter of oxygen. So, the more breath, the more calories we burn.
- Raises the body's inner heat, making cells more pliable, allowing intercellular fluids to circulate, carrying nutrients in and toxins out.

4—Your Main Excretory System

- Eliminates waste that slows you down and makes you sick.
- Breath activates the diaphragm, which in turn stimulates the lymphatic system to remove more toxins.
- Breath massages the lymph nodes, the body's sewer system, double the size of the circulatory system. Lymph carries away the dead white blood cells, toxins and other waste.
- Unlike blood pumped by the heart, lymph travels only by breath and the body's natural movements.
- 70 percent of the body's waste is swept out on the exhale as a gas.

- Deep belly breathing can increase the body's pace of waste elimination by 15 times!
- Shallow breathing forces the body to store waste, as fat.

Blood transports nutrients and oxygen to the cells. The cells then excrete debris and toxins into the lymphatic system, where waste is deactivated and eventually returned to the blood system, to run through the kidneys and liver for a good cleaning.

Poor breathing and lack of movement leads to slow lymph. Slow lymph leads to slow removal and cleaning of toxins from the blood, which in turns makes us ripe for illness, weight gain, fatigue and high blood pressure. Breathe deeply and keep your sewers active!

5—Your Life Force

Your breath is a gift.
The first sign of life. The hello cried at birth.
The last sign of life. The goodbye gasped at death.

- We need breathe more than food or water.
  How many weeks can you live without food? Four to six weeks. How many days can you live without water? Four to six days. How many minutes can you live without your breath? Six minutes. So, what is the most important fuel for your life?
- We breathe an average of 15 times each minute, or more than 23,000 times per day.
- Holding the breath is a way of focusing the energy. Have you noticed how weight lifters hold their breath? Olympic runners report that after reaching their peak speed, they hold their breath. Clench your fists or jaw, and notice how you hold your breath, to concentrate your energy. Remember stubbing your toe, and without thinking, you grabbed the toe and held your breath? In basic terms, this act was a form of healing, using *Pranic* energy stored in your body and transferred through your hands.

- How fully and how often we breathe influences our very life span. The ancient sages or *Rishis* of India taught that each person was born with a finite amount of breath, and when it was used up, life ended. This belief is supported by respiration studies. Rabbits, birds and dogs were categorized as rapid breathers, and had shorter life spans than those creatures observed with slow rates of breathing, such as tortoises and elephants.

Slow, deep breathing is better for maintaining the health of the heart than the fast, gasping breath of someone uptight and anxious. The deep breath truly feeds the muscles and systems of the body, assuring a robust and dynamic well-being.

Have you noticed when you are excited or anxious, your breathing is more like panting? Breathing from the neck and throat only, we rob ourselves of so much support. Often, I have Yoga students who begin to recognize, through practicing Yoga that they reserve deep breathing for rare events, such as Saturday mornings when their schedules are more relaxed. Don't pant your way through life.

Chapter 5

Yoga Breathing Exercises a.k.a. *Pranayama*

> *"Breath is aligned to both body and mind and it alone can bring them together."*
>
> Thich Nhat Hahn

From the ancient civilization of India, we have received the extraordinarily timeless practice of finely tuned breathing exercises or *Pranayama*.

A combination of two Sanskrit words: *Prana* meaning life force and *ayama*, expansion or exercise, *Pranayama* is much more than simply breathing. *Pranayama* is the method yogis use to reach higher levels of energy and awareness. As Pam Grout rightly titled her book on breathing, focused breathing will <u>Jump Start Your Metabolism</u>.

Noisy, chattering Yoga students are instantly quieted by a good teacher who asks, —Why are you wasting your *Prana*?‖ Besides decreasing our levels of useless chatter to conserve energy, adopting a breathing practice greatly improves awareness and focus.

Conserving and utilizing our life force is a central aspect of a sound Yoga practice. Various Yoga techniques can be employed for increasing, reducing and balancing our *Prana* and states of consciousness, including how we hold our breath.

Four aspects of breath are associated with yoga breathing exercises: inhaling, holding the inhaled breath, exhaling and holding after the exhaled or external breath is released. Retaining or holding inhaled breath is considered by some the real power, as it concentrates the life force and can transport the practitioner to a more subtle field of consciousness.

In my classes, I like to direct the students' attention to the holds between the inhale and the exhale, and the exhale and the inhale. I refer to these moments as a *pause*.

We inhale a full breath. We pause.
We exhale a full breath. We pause.

How do you feel in the first pause? Full of air, is it difficult to stay still, do you want to exhale?

How do you feel in the second pause? Without air, are you anxious, do you want to gulp air?

Amazingly, students report finding calm and peace in the pauses. They realize there is nothing to do, no action required. Rather, they can experience what it is like to have no breath or plenty of breath, to live without or with. And they find contentment in both states.

In combination with poses, breathing exercises can restore one's sense of vitality and energy, releasing feelings of fatigue and imbalance. Whether due to exercise, sleep, eating or mental and emotional exhaustion, a worn out and worn down feeling can be reversed with regular Yoga breathing.

Let's go to the BAR...Breathe And Relax.

BASIC GUIDELINES FOR PRACTICING YOGA BREATHING

1. While counterintuitive, begin with a full exhalation. Until the lungs are completely empty, a full inhale can't occur.

2. Unless congested, breathe through the nose only. The nostrils and respiratory system are all tangled up with the nervous system, and by restricting inhales and exhales to the nose, we deepen our relaxation. Nose breathing utilizes and strengthens the abdominal muscles, directing and pulling more air and thus more oxygen into the lower lobes of the lungs, where the greatest potential of oxygen exchange occurs. Further, the nose protects us from inhaling impurities and the mouth from drying out. (Watch a newborn, it naturally breathes only through the nose. Like becoming fearful, mouth- breathing is a learned skill, and is often

associated with fear or some other stressor that makes us need more air, faster.)

3. When an exercise calls for retaining the breath, if retention or exhalation is tough, reduce the duration of the inhale. Retention is how we charge the body. Never hold the breath longer than comfortable.

4. For optimum health, make the exhale twice as long as the inhale, to empty the body of toxins, wastes and poisons. Scuba divers are taught to hold the breath four times as long as the length of their inhale.

5. Practice on an empty stomach, at least four hours after eating. Smoking is not a complimentary practice for optimum health, and should be discontinued.

6. Sit upright and comfortably, if possible, in a clean and quiet, well ventilated, private space. Slumped posture and tight clothes restrict the lungs from fully inflating. Don't sabotage yourself, create good conditions.

7. Most teachers advise against practicing Yoga Breathing when sick or with a fever. When sick, relax and be aware of the breath; that is enough.

TO WARM UP, OBSERVE NATURAL BREATHING

1. With eyes closed, sit comfortably or lie on your back, and become aware of your breath. Like slowing down our turbo-gobbling at the dinner table, establishing a more relaxed, soothing rate of breathing requires awareness.

2. Concentrate on the nostrils, the rings around the nostrils and the small triangular area above the upper lip. See if you can feel the bare, natural breath. Don't force or try to regulate your breathing, just observe it. *This exercise is part of the phenomenal technique taught at Vipassana Meditation Centers, see Chapter 6 on Meditation.*

3. Can you feel the temperature of your breath? Cool going in, warmer coming out?

4. Can you feel which nostril is inhaling and exhaling?

5. Continue to watch your breath and what happens to your body as you breathe. Become aware of the throat, the chest and lungs, feeling the ribcage move.

6. Can you feel your abdomen rise and fall with your inhale and exhale?

7. Connect the entire experience, from your nostrils to your belly, and enjoy this free fill up of the life force.

TO WARM UP, PRACTICE PROPER NOSE BREATHING

1. Sit, inhale normally through your nose, mouth closed. Place lightly clasped hands over belly.

2. As you exhale through your nose, slightly tighten your throat, as if quietly snoring.

3. Notice you must contract your abdominal muscles to make the ―snoring‖ sound on exhale. The tighter you contract your stomach muscles, the louder the exhaled snoring sound. If you can make the noise, you are breathing properly.

4. Once you can make this sound with a shallow breath, increase the depth of each breath while making a resonant snoring sound with each exhale. For fun, add the noise on inhale. The use of the abdominal muscles is why this is called abdominal breathing.

5. Practice this type of breathing lying down, sitting and walking, with or without the sound, until it is second nature. Routinely breathe through the nose, especially when exhaling while exercising, with or without noise.

ELEVATOR BREATH

1. Sit, close your eyes and fully empty your lungs. Imagine a slow moving elevator that travels up and down your spine, powered by your breath.

2. Check in with yourself and determine what type of energy you need at this moment. Could you use some heavenly inspiration from above to motivate you? Or do you need to feel grounded, to have the support of the solid earth below for footing? Depending on what you need, you will either begin inhaling from the crown of your head downward, or from the tailbone upward.

3. Inhale fully, moving your elevator along the spine from high to low or from low to high. Feel free to visualize your elevator, maybe it is all crystal or gold.

4. Slowly exhale through the nose, moving your elevator back to its starting position.

5. Continue to move your elevator up or down the spine on the inhale. Return the elevator to its starting position on the exhale. Practice for five or more breaths, up to three times a day.

ELEVATOR BREATH VARIATION

Follow all the instructions above, but direct your awareness to counting the number of seconds you are able to inhale. I like to say mentally, ―One hippopotamus, two hippopotamus‖ as a way of measuring the seconds. Whatever you get for your inhale, be it three or five or seven hippos, make sure your exhale is longer and slower. So, if you inhale for 8 seconds, make your exhale 12 or more seconds long. And remember, a relaxed human being can inhale for 22 seconds! So when you are tense, count your hippopotamuses, and see if you can't lengthen your breath.

OUR BREATHING IS HIGHLY STRUCTURED AND POWERFUL

When breathing according to our design, human beings inhale and exhale through primarily one nostril at a time. In other words, one nostril will be open and the other partially blocked. Approximately every 90 to 110 minutes, the body automatically switches the primary nostril, and the opposite or alternate nostril takes over for another 90 to 110 minutes. Throughout the day and night, when we are in good health, this alternation in breathing occurs.

However, when the body is not in top form, due to poor health, environmental problems, emotional upheaval, diet or inadequate exercise, natural rotation in the breath may not occur. One nostril will become dominant, which means the two sides of the brain are getting uneven amounts of oxygen. The longer the body relies on one nostril only, the more at risk we are for getting sick. Yogis teach that more than one day---24 hours---of single nostril breathing is another flashing light on our dashboard that warns, —check engine."

For example, when we sleep on our right side, we breathe through the left nostril only. If we don't switch sides during the night, the right nostril, and subsequently, the left brain, is not stimulated.

To adjust or correct for this problem and others, Yoga offers countless breathing exercises. *Alternate Nostril Breathing* is used to balance nostril switching, restore the body's equilibrium and sense of well-being.

As you prepare to enter into the world of yoga breathing exercises, take a moment to center yourself with a bit of reflection or meditation. *See Chapter 6 on Meditation.*

TREES AS LUNGS MEDITATION

Sit comfortably, eyes closed. Imagine you are either sitting or lying down under a favorite tree. See the tree solidly rooted yet flexible in the wind, able to move easily with the breath of the breeze. Appreciate your beautiful, full tree that provides shade and shelter. See the tree as an extra set of lungs for you, functioning outside your body. See your exhale drifting upward to feed the trees. Inhale, enjoying the awareness that the tree is serving you breakfast, then taking your breath away. Experience the full harmonious circle of breathing, the conspiracy (Latin meaning *to breathe with or together*) between you and the tree.

Breathing exercises should be done in the order provided, and can be done alone or with seated poses interspersed between the individual breathing exercises. If you do poses between breathing exercises, repeat or hold each posture for the equivalent of four times or four breaths.

Calming Breath

To calm down and center ourselves. Inhale fully. Loudly say the *O* of the *Om* for 50 percent of the exhale and the *Mmmm* for the other 50 percent. Repeat for five breaths.

Bellows Breath

Two minutes of amplified, normal nose breathing. Imagine your breath is following a garland from the top of your head (crown *chakra*) down the front of the body to the end of the spine (root *chakra*.) *To learn about chakras, see end of this chapter.* At the root *chakra*, begin to exhale up the garland on the back of the body, ending at the crown and begin again. If you wish to draw energy from the earth, begin the inhale at the root *chakra*, coming up the garland to the crown, with exhale going down back to root *chakra* and begin again. This breath can be gradually speeded up, and the length of time increased from two minutes, to fan the heat or fire. After each forceful exhale immediately inhale a breath of equal duration. At first, do eight or 10 breaths, which constitute one round. Build up to five rounds.

Like the blacksmith's bellows, *Bellows Breath* heats up and stimulates energy, toning the abdomen, massaging the internal organs and stimulating the lymph system.

Shining Skull

Get moving without an alarm clock, coffee or sugar! Regular practitioners of *Shining Skull* radiate good health, as the breath cleanses and energizes the entire system. Shining Skull is a conscious experience opposite of normal breathing. Normal breathing involves active inhalation and passive exhalation; this practice is the reverse. Shining Skull:

- Cleanses the nasal passages, lungs and entire respiratory system.
- Strengthens and increases the capacity of the lungs and ribcage muscles.
- Helps drain the sinuses and eliminate accumulated mucus.
- Removes bronchial congestion. Over time, asthma is relieved and virtually eliminated. *Do not do during an asthma attack.*

- Helps remove large quantities of carbon monoxide, permitting the red blood cells to take on more oxygen.
- Massages stomach, liver, spleen, heart and pancreas.
- Improves digestion.
- Refreshes and invigorates the mind, sending a shot of oxygen to the frontal lobes of the brain.
- Creates a feeling of exhilaration.
- Increases the supply of stored life energy.

Can your alarm clock or candy bar do all that? Close your eyes and mouth, breathe only through nose. Take a few deep breaths to prepare. As you exhale, imagine you are snuffing a fly or butterfly off your nose. The forced exhale feels like a short burst of breath, causing your abdominal muscles to contract briefly and your diaphragm to move down. Optionally, place your hands on your belly, and feel your stomach pumping or jumping quickly.

No inhale action is required; the vacuum created automatically pulls in air, called passive breathing. Repeat snuffing and pumping, one exhale per second. Start with three rounds of 20 to 30 pumpings. Gradually increase to 60 pumpings, one minute.

Three Locks

Exhale fully, lock throat by tucking chin down to chest, Suck in belly, locking naval. Consciously pull up and —lock‖ rectum. Hold breath, then unlock rectum, naval, chin and inhale. Repeat. Pulls and redirects energy toward the spine. Mastery of this breathing exercise will cause total realignment of all body systems, as well as activate spiritual and mental awakening.

Fire Essence Breath

Exhale and tuck chin against neck/chest in chin lock. Rapidly pump the belly inside, contracting and expanding abdominal muscles. Try three rounds of 10 pumpings per round, to start. Inhale and exhale after each round. Build up to 60-100 pumpings per round. Cleans up digestive orders, constipation, strengthens abdomen. Best done when stomach and bowels are empty. *Do not do if more than three months pregnant.* Excellent after delivery, to tighten up pelvic and abdominal muscles. Proven to help flatten the abdomen.

Furnace Breath

Inhale making soft snoring noise in throat, like a baby sleeping. Swallow to hold breath for up to 10 counts. Exhale from left nostril only, holding right closed with right thumb. Do eight complete cycles. Removes phlegm from throat and improves digestion.

Alternate Nostril Breathing

Hold right hand up to nose, with elbow slightly tucked to your side and shoulder relaxed. Left hand rests on thigh. Gently close right nostril with right thumb and inhale from the left. Close left nostril with ring finger and exhale from right. Keep left nostril closed and inhale from right. Close right nostril with thumb and exhale from left.

These steps comprise one round. Retention of breath can be added between each inhale and exhale, to promote the development of muscle mass. When practicing to relieve anxiety, concentrate on soft and slow breath.

Moon and Sun, Cooling and Heating Breaths

Cooling Moon Breath: With right hand, use thumb to close right nostril and ring finger to close left. Inhale through left and exhale through right, repeatedly. Useful during warm weather or when the body feels warm, as it is cooling.

Heating Sun Breath: With right hand, use thumb to close right nostril and ring finger to close left. Inhale through right and exhale through left, repeatedly. Especially good in cold weather and when you need to feel warm.

A Tiny Primer on Chakras

So, just what are the chakras? From a Yoga perspective, the nervous system is roughly referenced as the six *Chakras* (seventh above the body, the crown *chakra*). Chakras are closely associated with the glands.

The word *Chakra* translates from the Sanskrit as *wheel* or *vortex*, an energy center linked to the brain, through the spinal column. Regarded as a center or seat of consciousness, each *Chakra* operates in a clockwise action as a switching station for a specific function of the brain.

Chakra 7—The Crown

Governs cortex, administers all spiritual, mental and physical activities. Associated with clear knowing.

Chakra 6—The Third Eye (above eyes, center of forehead)

Governs consciousness, assimilates nervous stimulation and sends to brain. Associated with clairvoyance. The top of the nervous system is just below this area, at the top of the nasal passages.

Chakra 5—The Throat

Governs respiration, vocalization and tongue. Controls saliva and bronchia. Associated with communication, speaking your truth.

Chakra 4—The Heart

Governs heart and circulation, electromagnetically charges the blood and body fluids, including lymph. Associated with love and realizing Oneness. The bridge chakra, connecting the three lower chakras, more associated with the physical world and the three upper chakras, more associated with the spiritual world.

Chakra 3—The Solar Plexus

Governs stomach, spleen, pancreas, liver, gall bladder and kidneys. Controls secretion of hormones and digestive acids. Associated with power and control and one's identity.

Chakra 2—The Sacral

Governs intestines, reproductive functions, pregnancy. Associated with physical desires and appetites, including sexuality and reproduction.

Chakra 1—The Root or Base

Governs bladder, rectum, and parts of nervous system. Associated with survival and shelter, basic needs. The last three inches of the elimination system is also the end of our nervous system, where the sphincter is tucked up next to the tailbone.

The ultimate goal of Yoga, when practiced in the purest sense, is to awaken dormant energy coiled at the lowest or root *Chakra*, and lead it upward to unite with the higher Supreme consciousness, accessed through the seventh or crown *Chakra*. This stored divine energy at the base of the spine is called *Kundalini*.

Yoga study is fascinating and illuminating; for example, each chakra is also associated with a sound and a color. <u>Do Chair Yoga</u> is an introductory text, inviting the reader to become a student of Yoga. For more instruction and knowledge, see the work of Swami Sivananda and Swami Vishnudevananda.

Rolled Pipe Tongue Cooling Breath

Roll tongue like a pipe, stick out of mouth and inhale, drawing air over tongue. If you can't roll your tongue, this is actually an inherited talent, do *Hissing Breath*: Slightly open mouth, with teeth slightly parted and tongue planted behind lower teeth and inhale. For both styles of cooling breath, after inhaling, swallow and exhale through left nostril, holding right nostril closed with right thumb. Repeat five to eight times. Helps when you are hungry or thirsty and no food or water are available.

Humming Bee Breath

Three fingers placed not pressed on eyeballs, index fingers pointed up toward hairline, thumbs in ears. Inhale. On the exhale say *Om*, with five percent of the exhaled sound *O* of the *Om* and 95 percent of the exhaled sound the *M*. Concentrate on third eye and crown *chakra*. This sounds like a powerful bee has taken over the inside of the head. To reincarnate as a bee in India must be bliss, hovering over the mango flowers. (I think the Humming Bee sounds more like a giant truck blasting its horn to warn of a head on collision.) Rather like the trusty aspirin in terms of its versatility, Humming Bee Breath helps with anger, anxiety, arthritis, asthma, backache, blood pressure (regulating high and low), colds, depression, dizziness, fatigue, hair loss, indigestion, insomnia, paralysis and stroke, PMS, pregnancy and thyroid.

Chapter 6

Meditation: Slow Down, Live Long

Man goes into the noisy crowd
To drown his own clamor of silence.
                                    Rumi

From the Hindu tradition, Swami Rama said, —We are taught now to move and behave in the external world, but we are never taught how to be still and examine what is within ourselves. At the same time, learning to be still and calm should not be made a ceremony or part of any religion; it is a universal requirement of the human body. When one learns to sit still, he or she attains a kind of joy that is inexplicable. The highest of all joys that can ever be attained or experienced by a human being can be attained through meditation. All of the other joys in the world are transient and momentary, but the joy of meditation is immense and everlasting.‖

—Many of us spend a great deal of time in inane conversation because we are so frightened of and feel so socially awkward in the silent spaces. We fear silence when we are alone as well, and so we often live with a constant background of radio chat shows or muzak,‖ wrote Father John Main, the founder of the World Community for Christian Meditation (www.wccm.org) —In meditation we cross the threshold from background noise into silence. This is vital for us because silence is necessary if the human spirit is to thrive and to be creative.‖

To better explain the <u>Dhammapada</u>, Buddha's teachings, a story is told to illustrate the importance of self care through meditation. Buddha was dying, and his disciples were gathering to spend time at his deathbed. A monk named Attadattha decided not to join the group, and instead went to his cell to meditate. When the other monks tattled to Buddha, Buddha praised

Attadattha's conduct, explaining that one's spiritual welfare should not be abandoned for the sake of others.

Like listening to the quiet mystery of a shell held to the ear, meditation allows us to deepen down into the inner, peaceful place within. When we set aside time for silence, we enter a well or web that unites and holds us all.

Yoga and meditation produce deep relaxation, resting our bodies at a cellular level. The first thing my massage teacher, Dr. Nedungadi V. Haridas of Chennai says to every patient he sees, is, —Don't worry. Just don't worry.‖ Relaxation is one of our best antidotes for worry. For so many of us, our choices for relaxation actually can increase our worries!

How many of us relax curling up with a bag of salty or sugary snacks to watch a television program laced with violence? True relaxation does not involve potato chips or blood samples, but quiet stillness. Our bodies yearn for a technology free zone, with no greasy refreshments served.

Even joggers seeking the benefits of exercise can't hear the birds, paying attention to ipod tunes.

Too noisy, too busy, we do less and less self care.

Inviting friends to visit the School of Ancient Wisdom in Bangalore for a weekend retreat, I found no takers. —Life is really busy, life is full, life is crazy, work is wild, no time for time off, would love to but not this year, swimming rough financial waters.‖ My email inbox is full of people longing to be set free, trapped by their own design. If they only knew the warden is in the mirror.

Sadly, I have received near identical responses from friends in the US, when I have invited them for a relaxing time at my Northern Vermont home, Shantivanam, the Peace Forest.

—I feel like I am becoming mentally ill and my husband says he doesn't even know if he likes me anymore, but I just can't schedule any time away right now.‖

Mortgages, loans and other weighty debt are driving us to push faster and faster, avoiding relaxation and rejuvenation.

I remember meeting Lily Anna Sophia Nutt, a grand older woman with an adorable house in Ann Arbor, Michigan. It was 1971; I was in my sophomore year at the University of Michigan, and needed money. I answered Lily's add for a girl to weed her garden and do other odd jobs, as assigned. Lily was still recovering from her husband's recent and untimely (what a concept) death.

—Jim retired from the hardware store and I gave him a wonderful party. He ate a big steak and died that night at the party.‖ Lily had been waiting for the travel retirees grant themselves, particularly men whose life is defined by constantly working.

Sr. Joan Chittister, the courageous prophet in America's Roman Catholic Church, says women's rights will become a reality when men realize the price they pay for the uneven balance of power. Expecting men to become mega earners exacts a great toll on their hearts and health.

My husband, a physician who retired from medicine when it stopped being a service and became a business, says we would all do each other a favor if we stated the true causes of death. Rather than listing heart disease, cancer, stroke and diabetes, he says we need to state the truth: cigarettes, alcohol, diet, stress and lack of exercise.

Full of anxiety and dissatisfaction, we can easily slip into the grip of a variety of addictive behaviors, which promise instant yet impermanent distraction from that inner sense of discontent. Gambling, promiscuity, overeating/drinking/drugging and the perennial favorite, shopping, buy us little long term relief.

At Ayurvedic massage school in Neyyer Dam, Kerala, I met a young Yoga teacher from England. I asked if she had taught Yoga for long. —No, I quit a job with a large grocery store network in London, I couldn't do it anymore.‖

—What couldn't you do?‖ I asked.

—I created the circulars that went in the newspapers every week, describing our specials. Basically, my message was always the same; _You aren't a good mother if you don't buy this item.' I couldn't do it anymore, pushing compulsive shopping.‖

Well, she may have stopped being the messenger, but the message lives on, through advertisements, commercials, and billboards. Much of the world economy is based on this message.

How crazy is it to work hard selling stuff so we can buy some other stuff someone else is working hard to sell?

SIMPLE VERSUS SOPHISTICATED

Outside my window in Bangalore, when Narayan the gardener is working with his little boy, Nagesh, I feel like the paparazzi, stalking them with fascination. Hauling the heavy hose, squatting to plant or water, pruning the scrubs, trimming the dead palm fronds, Narayan is in motion. In India, at more than one garden, I have watched squatting men cut their lawns with hand clippers. Dry leaves are swept off the lawns with three foot tall monkey grass brooms, requiring the sweeper to work with a bent back. In other words, gardeners in India practice Yoga daily.

I once watched Narayan at dusk, running with his gleeful son in his arms, to turn off a hose. He ran for several minutes, the child jubilant. Another afternoon I saw Narayan sitting under a small tree with his sleeping baby in his lap, lightly patting the boy's chest. Catching my eye with his smile, Narayan sat. Tears flooded my vision. What a lucky son and father. Working and living simply, with time to enjoy the sun and each other.

At meal time, fruit peels are carefully set aside by Narayan's family. Later, they are lovingly given to our cow, Lakshmi.

Interspecies empathy, seeing the connections between all life forms, is essential not only for our peace of mind, but for the very survival of the planet. Bloodlust sports have led to a new crisis in the wild, where the traumatic experiences of witnessing the massacre of their families impairs the normal brain and behavior development of young elephants. Animal ethnologist Eve Abe of Uganda is working to build a community center to help both elephants and humans in their recovery from violence.

Why do we continually express surprise when we see such connections between ourselves and the forms of life with whom we share this spinning orb? Isn't all life just a soup of carbon, hydrogen, oxygen and nitrogen?

Though armed with every communications device we can invent and buy, many still feel disconnected from themselves and others. As this book heads for publication, I've just heard there are officially more cell phones than people on Planet Earth.

Listening to the news of something going on somewhere other than where we are, we have lost our place in the Present Moment, the only place we can be certain to find contentment.

Isn't it ironic? We want everything now, but we are living somewhere other than here. I would guess well over 90 percent of the phone calls I inadvertently overhear at the airport are minute-by-minute reports on where the caller is going and their estimated time of arrival. We are narrating, not living, our lives. The news is, we've become our own cable news channels, reporting traffic and weather on the eights or sevens or however often we call.

I met a man, when discussing the breakdown of his marriage, said he, —Didn't have the bandwidth to handle her.‖

What needs to change?

Plenty, and one of our humanity's strengths is that we can change.

In 1990, I decided to make a lifestyle change, that I was done seeking objects outside myself to be happy. I had been an unfaithful meditator for nine years. It was time to commit to meditation and find the health and peace within.

My friend Regis Cummings, a deacon at St. Augustine's Roman Catholic Church in Montpelier, Vermont, agreed to teach me how to meditate. We had been talking about his tutoring me for some time, and somehow the time never materialized.

Enjoying a quick lunch together at Angelino's Pizza Parlor, I again off-handedly asked, —When will you teach me meditation, Regis?

—Right now,‖ he answered. What a perfect introduction to this ancient tradition that crosses all faith traditions, nations and races. My first lesson included this powerful message, right at the top: you can meditate anywhere and at any time, in a plastic chair near the door in a pizza parlor, in the middle of the busy lunch hour.

Teaching Yoga one fall night in my town of Glover, Vermont, the class was comfortably settling into the final cool down phase of the evening, ready to enjoy silent meditation before heading home. Next door, a Truck full of firewood was being dumped. It sounded more like a train wreck than a wood delivery. Our first ―tsks‖ turned quickly to chuckles, as all present experienced the perfection of the moment: meditation requires no external conditions, for it is all about entering our inner world.

Following my first short silent meditation with Regis at Angelino's Pizza (doesn't that mean ―little Angel‖ in Italian? More of a sacred space than I thought?) I asked, ―How long will it be before I get it? My mind was so full of thoughts, it wasn't peaceful at all.‖

With all the honesty he could muster, Regis replied, ―Oh, if you're like me, about 10 years.‖ We laughed and he reminded me that the time and intention I brought to my meditation would determine the benefits. He encouraged me to meditate often, by myself as well as with others, and in one regular location as well as unfamiliar places. All of these efforts would deepen and broaden my practice.

Wanting to touch the bliss and peace of the Inner Bethany, I became especially diligent about attempting meditation in unlikely places. After all, if I could meditate at a soccer game or in an airport, perching on the pillow on my back porch would be a cinch, right?

Well, yes and no. Because more than outside noise, what influences our meditation, just like our Yoga and our life as a whole, is not so much what is going on *around us* as *in us*.

Like the friend who thinks moving to a new city will shake her depression and give her a fresh start, meditators learn that wherever you meditate, there you are. You, not the environment, are still the Key Factor. Yes, that is the good news and bad news.

My meditation with the World Community for Christian Meditation took me to India in 1998 on a pilgrimage for peace, co-led by the Dalai Lama, and again, with him on a pilgrimage to Northern Ireland in 2000, for the same purposes. My memories of meditating with Catholics and Protestants in the Belfast City Hall, where no Catholic had ever set foot until the Dalai Lama requested this as a condition of his visit, are sweet. More than 600 of us were breathing together, in that conspiracy of shared breath and silence.

Centering prayer, as taught by the Institute for Spiritual Development in Burlington, Vermont, and many other locations around the world, is a close cousin of Christian meditation. *See bibliography, M. Basil Pennington book.*

MANTRAS AND AFFIRMATIONS

Through Siddha Yoga (www.siddhayoga.org) and Sivananda Yoga (www.sivananada.org), I learned meditation using *Mantras*. A *Mantra* is a sound, word or series of both utilized by meditators as a sacred way to draw closer to the Divine. Whether you believe the Divine or God is within or without or above, the *Mantra* can serve as a passport.

Within the Christian tradition of meditation, traced back to the desert fathers, WCCM teaches the use of the prayer-phrase *Maranatha*. From the Old Testament, it means almost the same thing that *Namaste* does in Yoga, —I honor the God within.‖

Within the more secular world, affirmations are popular for meditation and to guide our daily thinking and actions, powerful thought patterns that affirm a positive belief. By mentally repeating an affirmation regularly with conviction, we shift our thinking and our actions to a healthy and optimistic course.

Affirmations are the best antidote for worry. Using our creative energy to repeat positive thoughts, we retrain our minds. When feeling swept up by worry, consciously choose worship instead, thinking thoughts of gratitude and hope. Choose faith, not fear. We repeat affirming thoughts silently, verbally and in writing.

A simple affirmation is, —I am safe. I am at peace and at one with all life.‖ We can write our own affirmations, by quietly sitting and phrasing our heart's desire in present tense, healthy terms. Metaphysical healer and author Louise Hay is a great resource in this area.

Of course, as with all human endeavors, intention is critical when meditating. And if we find ourselves calling out (chanting either mentally or audibly) the name of the Divine without being calm and centered, it is unlikely we will experience any response!

My most challenging and rewarding experience of group meditation was the Vipassana Meditation Course in Bangalore, 10 days of silence, 10 hours a day of seated meditation. (www.dhamma.org)

The entire course is based on the teachings of the Buddha, who taught meditation more than 2500 years ago. Like Buddha, Jesus also saw and taught the value of making time for silence. *And from time to time he would withdraw to lonely places for prayer. . . During this time he went out one day into the hills to pray, and spent the night in prayer to God. Luke 5:16; 6:12*

My first morning at the Vipassana course, I stood at sunrise, watching the red orb appear from behind the trees. My teacher, Lakshmiappana, came and said, ―I don't know what your practice is, but here I want you to look at nothing and think of nothing but your meditation. Keep your eyes downcast or closed at all times. Do not look at people or things. You will gain much.‖

―My practice?‖ I thought. ―I was just being human!‖ But I obeyed Lakshmiappana, and watched no sunrises or sunsets during the course, because I wanted the benefits.

Other course rules included no books, no writing, no Yoga, no speaking. We woke at 4 a.m. and retired at 9 p.m. I knew the 20 some other women I slept in the same room with, ate one meal a day in the same room with and meditated in the same room with by their shoes and coughs alone.

Within one hour of sitting down for our first meditation session on Day One, I heard Them, the backhoe, trucks and tractors. Outside our window in the dusty heat of Bangalore, the new meditation or Dhamma Hall was being built. Unlike so many other construction projects I had watched in this city, most of the work was being done with heavy equipment, not the usual dozens of men and women carrying baskets of dirt, bricks and cement block on their heads.

For 12 hours a day, every day, these diesel powered machines operated, right outside our small meditation hall. Our windows had no glass or screens. I was annoyed by the noisy busboy at the pizza parlor with Regis during my first meditation session. Could I handle earth-moving equipment?

At the close of the Vipassana course, I joked with my teacher who taught this Industrial Strength, turbo-charged course! What a blessing! By the third day I no longer heard the machines. By the fifth day the coughing, belching and knuckle cracking of my fellow meditators began to fade, as well.

Ultimately, the bigger irritant is always my own mind; those painful, shameful memories that float up in the silence. During Vipassana, a 10- year- old scene planted itself squarely in my lap. I flashed to a night I gossiped and joked in a restaurant about someone, only to learn at the end of the meal that his daughter was sitting in the booth behind me. Other times on my Vipassana perch, tears would run down my cheeks, silently releasing an ache I couldn't even name. I was being washed out.

Spending time with myself sitting on the pillow was something I quickly came to love at the Vipassana Course. I would wake before dawn and say to myself, ―Another Bethany Day! I can't even say _hello' or _thank you' to anyone, it is all about me!‖

Becoming comfortable with our own company and then going even beyond that, to discover just how much you have within to sustain yourself, is one of the great joys of meditating. Like Yoga, the benefits often appear after the practice.

Resisting a role or expectations, we can find incredible freedom in meditation. In fact, the ultimate goal as stated in Vipassana meditation is liberty, to be free of all suffering and misery. This emancipation is possible once we see that all of our suffering, which the Buddha called *Dukka*, is our own doing, created by our mind in its endless game of liking and disliking.

Discovering a reservoir of calm within, sensing everything is OK and in harmony, you are better prepared for the two-hour gridlock on the bridge or the oily stain on your favorite silk shirt. (Those stains will outlive us all.) While the link between meditation and its results might not be as obvious as Overeat and Get Fat, it is just as real. Through meditation, we find new ways to approach our anxieties, pain, fears and addictions, because we are learning to no longer live in reaction, in a knee jerk fashion to whatever is tossed our way.

Reviewing our day, it can seem we spent most of our waking hours in reaction. You answer the phone, the door, your children's questions. You explain your decisions to colleagues, your spouse, your former spouse, your children. You defend yourself, stand up for yourself, exhaust yourself.

When we live in a state of reaction, it is tiring and powerless. Others set our agenda and frame our day with their demands and requirements. As world-class Olympian reactors, we have a dangerous habit of forming an opinion about everything that happens. We like the weather. We don't like his haircut. We hate the traffic. We love ice cream. We detest the smell of the burning garbage. We love to hear good music. We can't bear the sound of planes overhead. And so on.

The sages teach that using our limited life energy or *Prana* to form, feel and express opinions on subjects that are impermanent is foolish. It is said everything is changing, everything is *Anicca*. If something is temporary and passing anyway, why are we bothering to judge it? Why not observe it dispassionately, and let it go? Why not see everything as changing? Why not find solace in knowing that whatever is bugging you, it too, shall pass?

Don't worry that you will become a lifeless zombie, disengaged from the moment. Express your joy! Enjoy the moment! Be in it, as opposed to evaluating it.

Likewise, even things we are thrilled with do not necessarily require our opinions and energy. If you are serious about wanting a balanced and even approach to the day, if you truly desire to feel at ease and level headed, then the whole habit of labeling likes and dislikes has to be abandoned. You are up to something larger, wanting to find a sense of peace and equanimity that is not driven by the weather or soup served at lunch. Rather, your well-being is centered within, in that inner place of silence and perfection that is not influenced by anything outside of you.

Once we stop playing the game called reaction, we can begin living a life of creation and responding. When we create and respond, we are making conscious choices about how we want to use our time and our talents. We are no longer standing on the other side of the net, returning someone else's serve.

See the word REACTION floating in space. Consciously move the letter C and put it at the front of the word. You are now in CREATION.

REACTION
...C...

CREATION

True joy or happiness or bliss, or as it is referred to in India, *Ananda*, is already within you. You don't need to add ice cream or a holiday in Bali to feel even happier. Think of a baby you tried to make laugh. Recall all those foolish faces and voices you showered on the infant, determined to get a smile and giggle to emerge. The smile and giggle is standard on the model called Human Being. We all come with it; we all carry it within us. But when we are so busy looking for smiles and giggles outside, and even busier identifying everything we like and dislike, we rarely make the time to go inside and find our bliss, our *Ananda*.

Meditation provides the key to this lovely interior space of joy and peace. By focusing our attention within (without technology or electricity) we can find our equilibrium.

Holding our attention is a job of the brain's right hemisphere, so meditating is actually great exercise for the brain. Researchers have shown that meditation alters brain patterns, creating new neuropathways and causing the cortex to grow thicker.

Studies show those who meditate 40 minutes a day actually increase the right hemisphere cortical regions related to touch, sound and sight. And the thickening of the frontal lobes also slows down the effects of aging, which means with meditation we become calmer and remain younger.

VARIETIES OF MEDITATION

Like finding your favorite way to host a surprise party or pack your suitcase, one's style of meditation is personal and discovered through experience.

If you need sensory stimulation to stay focused, you may like to try meditating with beads, as the rosary used in the Catholic tradition.

For those who are more auditory, repeating a *mantra* silently often works.

Vipassana focuses on observing the breath and the sensations felt on the body.

The Yoga tradition of meditation known as Concentrated Gazing involves staring at a candle or image about two to three feet away, without blinking. When the eyes tire, the yogi closes her eyes and continues to meditate on the image burned into her brain. When that image disappears, staring at the candle resumes. This is the pattern, bringing the mind back to the flame whenever thoughts arise.

Mahatma Gandhi spent much of his life in walking meditation. Whenever he put his foot down on the ground, he would silently say the word —Rama‖, or God. Observers said his gait was like no other; it appeared he was almost being pulled forward into his next step.

Whatever the meditation technique, the ground rules are essentially the same. Remember to create good conditions for yourself. If other people are around, let them know you will be meditating for 15 or 30 or 60 or whatever minutes, and ask not to be interrupted for a phone call, a visitor, or to find the mayonnaise in the refrigerator.

If you can meditate around the same time and in the same place daily, you have found the best way to train your mind. Like a monkey jumping from tree to tree, your mind can be quieted by the meditation routine you establish. A familiar pillow or shawl can assist in creating this state, as well.

Making a decision to be the master of your own mind, that is, to stop playing the game of reaction and enter *Samadhi*, a state of concentration, is a giant step toward true happiness. Developing your will power, learning to control your thinking, is considered the shortest route to true enlightenment, to becoming a *Swami*, in harmony with all. Meditation is a great tool for developing will power and control over the senses and the mind.

How To Meditate

- Sit comfortably with a straight back. Exhale deeply. Relax.
- Close your eyes and mouth, breathe through nose only, unless congested.
- Observe yourself as strong, yet relaxed.
- Silently, begin your practice, whether it is repeating your mantra, with or without beads, observing your breath or another meditation technique.
- As thoughts pop up, let them float by like clouds, requiring no energy or opinion.
- When you notice you are thinking, don't judge yourself, simply return to your practice, focusing on your object of concentration.
- Expect and imagine nothing, spiritual or otherwise. Just be in the stillness.

Guided Meditation

Sometimes beginners like to be led in a guided meditation, to help them calm down and enter a state of quiet. Youtube has many free centering visualizations and guided meditations.

Chapter 7

Digging Our Grave with Our Teeth

Perhaps if you achieve a proper, healthy diet you will be encouraged to tackle the other four principles of Yoga—exercise; breathing; relaxation and positive thinking and meditation.

The Yoga Cookbook

In the novel <u>The Kite Runner</u>, an American travels to Afghanistan after the Taliban takeover, and spends a night in the home of a very modest Afghani family. At dinner, he asks why the children are not at the meal. —Already eaten,‖ his host replies.

While eating, the guest spies the children staring at his fancy watch, which tells the time in multiple time zones. Appreciating their hospitality, he gives the children his watch, demonstrating the high tech features.

The next morning, seeing the watch on the floor, he realizes the children were intently watching his plate, not his watch, as he ate their meal.

I suspect many hungry children feel this way about their well-fed fellow citizens.

In his book <u>Being Peace</u>, Thich Nhat Hanh writes, —When we eat a piece of meat or drink alcohol, we can produce awareness that 40,000 children die each day in the third world from hunger and that in order to produce a piece of meat or bottle of liquor we have to use a lot of grain.‖ This Buddhist monk further suggests that if all of us would reduce our consumption of meat and alcohol by just 50 percent, the world hunger situation would totally change.

Eating more than our fair share is not only killing children in Africa and India and South and Central America and the Philippines, it is killing the well to do children too, both those who go to bed hungry and those who go to bed stuffed with junk food.

SLOW DOWN AND TASTE THE TOMATO

In 1972, while an undergraduate at the University of Michigan, I interviewed with a mother of two about a live-in nanny position. She was flushed, having just ridden her bike up the steep hill from town. —Have you ever tasted fresh tuna?‖ she said brightly, holding the butcher paper-wrapped package up like a trophy.

—Uh, no,‖ I said. Until that moment, I hadn't considered tuna could be anything other than in a can.

—Oh, it is exquisite. I'm grilling it tonight for dinner.‖

About a year later, I met an old chum coming out of the grocery store, cradling a paper bag of produce with great anticipation. —Making tomato soup tonight. Can't wait!‖ Another food that didn't come from a can?

Working at an outdoor food concession, I watched a hungry teenager treated to an unexpected plate of hot French fries. He had been talking at the counter with other boys, busy wolfing down their orders. Once served, he stared at his plate, making no move to begin. He continued to talk with his friends, slowly squirting ketchup on one crisp potato spear at a time. Like a wine tester, he began with a single sample on his tongue, judging each bite. When his pals had finished, he was half a plate behind, teaching all of us about savoring food.

In Angela's Ashes, Frank McCourt writes the same lesson, with his story of sharing a buttered boiled egg with his brothers. My mouth watered as I read it. I ate a boiled egg immediately.

In India, I've watched hungry children:

- Eat ever so slowly, perhaps savoring the meal, but also because their shrunken stomachs can't process much very fast
- Comb through the refuse on the railroad tracks, looking for something to eat, even an orange peel
- Grab 50 bananas off a stalk in a 10 second frenzy

On flights to India, I've watched very large passengers:

- Request seat belt extensions to accommodate their girth
- Have the flight attendant place the food tray on the passenger's belly, because there was no way to get the tray table flat
- Eat an entire airline dinner and then take another meal out of their carry on

EATING LIKE A YOGI

Yogic scriptures assert that all modern diseases will disappear, when one practices proper breathing and eats a proper diet.

At Sivananda Yoga teacher training, we were taught to eat slowly and taste the food, to chew thoroughly because the first stage of digestion begins in the mouth. The teeth bite and grind food into small particles, so the saliva can cover as much as possible. The molars further reduce the food to a fine paste. Saliva contains enzymes that break down starches and converts them into sugars for easy absorption into the digestive system.

We were also taught that, after a meal, the stomach should be half full with food, a quarter full of liquid and a quarter empty. When I first told my hungry husband this rule, he confessed, —I think I leave the table with my stomach 5/4s full!‖ I believe he speaks for most of us.

But just what kind of comfort is our comfort food providing? Assurance that we will surely fall ill and die young? As Swami Sivananda said of overeating, —Most of us dig our grave with our teeth.‖

Some of the expressions we use after a meal are most revealing. —I'm stuffed.‖ —I'm packed.‖ —I couldn't eat another thing.‖

Sadly, the popular remedy for stomach discomfort is to swallow something else—an antacid or other treatment for gas and bloating. Some commercials advise taking such a product in advance of the meal, which means overeating is planned! Premeditated suicide?

A morbidly obese friend of mine once told me that she finally had figured out what her health problem was: —My doctor told me my heart was too small for my body.‖

Could she not remove the ever-so-thin veil he had courteously hung across her eyes? Do we really think toting around more weight than our joints and organs were intended to support won't result in disastrous consequences?

While visiting the Sri Aurobindo Ashram in Pondicherry, Tamil Nadu, India, I stayed at an international guesthouse. Most of the visitors were European and American. As fate would have it, every time I turned around I bumped into a large, blond American woman. Like me, she had no trouble expressing herself. She was particularly uninhibited, and regarded any person standing still as a target for conversation.

—I can't believe it!‖ she exclaimed in the dining room to breakfast wait staff, —I've learned I can't eat sugar, pickles, apples, beets, wheat and nuts. I just can't believe it, but that's what this doctor told me.‖

At noon, sitting in another dining room in the city, I found her across from me, again embarking on her long list of forbidden foods. —I can't have that, or this, or them, or those,‖ she continued, with more than an edge of anxiety.

Her harangue haunted me. Days later, I told Renu, my traveling companion, —I have thought a lot about that lady and her dietary restrictions. I know what I want to say to her now.‖

—What?‖ Renu asked.

—I would look at her and say, ‗Well, perhaps if you can't eat all these things, it's because other people need to.'‖ I would also suggest that, to maintain optimum health, we all

- Eat only when hungry at regular meal times. Swami Sivananda cautioned his disciples about false hunger. —The gastric fire is God. Wait for the appearance of this God within and only then offer Him some food.‖
- Don't snack between meals, become a slave to food or drink, eat late or when angry. Eating after sunset is unwise.

- Eat a fresh plant diet (fruits, vegetables, grains and beans), loaded with vitamins, minerals, phytochemicals, antioxidants and carotenoids, all immunity boosting compounds. Food that is closest to the sun (instead of going to a factory for processing) is best.
- Consume no artificial sweeteners, in beverages or food. These products are known to kill rats and change brain chemistry. Studies link them to neurological disorders, problems with vision and hearing, depression and memory. Many individuals diagnosed with fibromyalgia, MS and lupus may be suffering from methanol toxicity, caused when ingested sweetener reaches body temperature. Above 86 degrees Fahrenheit, the wood alcohol in the sweetener becomes formaldehyde and formic acid, causing metabolic acidosis, poisoning the body.
- Drink close to one quart of water daily for every 50 pounds of body weight.
- Consume foods with the lowest amounts of saturated fat and cholesterol. Choose only polyunsaturated fat. Known as the Good Fat, it stays liquid or soft at room temperature, like safflower and sunflower oils. Good fat is also found in seafood. Monounsaturated fats are also okay, such as olive and peanut oils.
- Limit saturated fats, found in animal sources, which typically remain solid at room temperature, such as butter and red meat.
- Avoid alcohol and caffeine.

My personal short set of diet rules goes like this: no wheat, no meat, no sweet, no grease, no greased lightning (alcohol). I also choose not to eat after 6 p.m., because most of those calories go directly to my storage units. And because I still am in my human form, I am able to adhere to this plan 80 percent of the time.

CHAPTER 8

CONSTIPATION: LEAVE IT BEHIND YOU

"How is your elimination?"
Yoga wellness questionnaire

Constipation may be the cause of all your problems. Is it time you allowed your body to let go, to naturally empty itself of all waste, impurities, defilements and everything else you are holding onto that no longer serves you?

Besides the incredible discomfort of irregularity, blocked bowels put us at risk for serious health problems. Many yogis believe constipation is the cause of virtually every problem that hits the human body, including paralysis and stroke. Storing toxins and waste the body has decided must be cast off is dangerous. Not only are you what you eat, you are what you store.

The formal medical term for being seriously constipated is autointoxication, self-poisoning caused by endogenous microorganisms, metabolic wastes, or other toxins produced within the body. Also known as autotoxemia, the symptoms include muddy thinking, short temper, poor decision-making, bad reflexes, bad breath, low energy and agitation.

Unfortunately, many of us, out of impatience, ignorance and desperation, resort to harsh and unnecessary chemical laxatives to force our bowels into action. Over time, such extreme measures take a toll on our finely tuned body, and naturally managed regularity becomes even more difficult to achieve. Some laxative manufacturers claim upwards of 80 percent of women are constipated.

Enemas and suppositories are far gentler, but again, unless used sparingly, they sabotage whatever training you are trying to give your Inner Pony. Becoming dependent on anything other than the easy functioning of a healthy system is most unwise, and, pun intended, it bites you in the butt.

A close friend was once vacationing far from home, and constipation was her constant companion. Panicked, she bought two enema kits and hid them under her seat on the tour bus, looking forward to some relief later at the hotel. During the day of frequent stops and starts, her bag of unusual souvenirs slid to the back of the bus. You can guess the rest of the story, the bus driver announcing on his microphone, —Will the person who left a bag of two enema kits pick them up at the front of the bus?‖

We tend to be easily embarrassed when the subject is elimination. In India, Ayurvedic physicians ask openly about bowel habits. Far from a topic to avoid, its influence is widely regarded and heeded. Our bodies are marvelously made, and made to work for years and years. When a function as key and routine as moving the bowels becomes impaired, we must pay attention.

I've had friends who've ended up in the emergency room with impacted bowels, even after self-administered but failed enemas, laxatives and the like. Like Yoga, there is no short cut to success. Regular practice is the only sure way to mastery.

YOUR CONSTITUTION IS A BIG DETERMINANT

My father likes to brag about the number of times a day he enters the —throne room‖, to evacuate his bowels. For those around him who experience this effort much less frequently and with more difficulty, his boasting is annoying.

How much credit can he really take for so successfully making daily donations to the bowl?

How much must we praise his genetic makeup, his constitution, for this ease of letting go?

Within Ayurvedic medicine, we are taught that there are three basic constitutions or body types: *Vata, Pitta* and *Kapha*. Called the three *Doshas*, most people have some aspect or qualities of each of the three within them, but rarely is someone evenly balanced. Ayurveda teaches that essentially, any internal pain we suffer is related to a constitutional imbalance.

Learning a bit about our unique nature, we can better select our diet and the Yoga poses most suited for us.

All living things have one or more *Dosha*, which are comprised of different arrangements of the five elements or energies that make up life: water, air, space, fire and earth. Examining a single cell, from an Ayurvedic viewpoint, the outer wall of the cell or structure is associated with *Kapha (water/earth)*; the center is associated with energy or *Vata (space/air)* and what is in between is the chemical activity, or *Pitta (fire/water)*.

From a most basic standpoint, *Vata* controls what is called the wind in the body, the movement like bowels, blood, breath, thoughts. When a *Vata* type gets sick, they usually find their vulnerability lies in what we call the mental area, insomnia, depression, panic attacks; their minds race and bowels stop. Vata body type is generally on the slim side and small boned.

Pitta is associated with fire or metabolism, that means digestion and when disordered, inflammation and infection. *Pitta* is often the *Dosha* of those body types of medium build, with freckles, red hair and short tempers.

Kapha is the more inert of the three, associated with structure, bones, phlegm and the waterlogged part of our being. When out of balance, *Kapha* leads to the flu, sinus trouble, weight gain. Procrastination and being slow to take action is also a *Kapha* quality. When a person has big wrists and ankles, we call them big boned, a sure sign of *Kapha* presence.

When determining body type, a general rule involves measuring bone size by wrapping one hand around the other wrist. If thumb overlaps fingers, Vata. If fingers touch, Pitta. If fingers don't meet, Kapha.

With this simple understanding, we can conclude that constipation is essentially a sign that *Vata* is out of balance. Beyond just reviewing one's own body type and tendencies toward disease, we can also learn our *Dosha* by listening to our pulses, the three point Ayurvedic way.

With your right hand, wrap your three fingers around your wrist. You will feel the pulse. Each finger represents a *Dosha*. The index finger is where the *Vata* pulse is felt. The middle finger for *Pitta* and the ring finger for *Kapha*.

By determining where the pulse feels the strongest, you identify the predominant *Dosha*. A throbbing index finger means *Vata* is strong. Check *Pitta* next, lift the index finger up and feel underneath the middle finger. If it is stronger than the *Vata* pulse, you are probably *Pitta* or *Kapha* dominant, or a combination.

Determining *Doshas* is tricky, as a strong pulse can also mean an imbalance in a particular *Dosha*.

It is common to have more than one *Dosha* operating in our body and even to have them change somewhat over our lifetime.

As you get into the habit of checking these pulses, you may notice changes in their strength, which can be an indication of imbalance or illness. For the constipated, *Vata* is always strong.

THE STORY YOUR BOWELS TELL

Just as we each have an individual, personalized understanding of our favorite food or meal, we also have unique experiences of constipation.

Deciding to end constipation, you begin a wonderful adventure with your body, an opportunity to get to know yourself from, literally, the inside out. Don't get caught up in thinking this is ―gross or unpleasant;‖ that is actually part of your problem. Until you accept elimination as a natural part of being you, it will remain a problem.

Your goal is bowels that function easily, reliably, painlessly, fully. I suspect you would like to know when and where you will have one or more daily movements. One family member has always seemed stunned by the sudden knock, knocking, knocking on her rectum door. Typically, we are at the grocery store when the urge hits her, immediately and insistently. ―It's now!‖ she whispers wide-eyed, bolting for the dirty bathroom for employees only. Knowing where all the public toilets are in her circle of travel is essential.

The Indian toilet, squatting over a hole rather than sitting on a tall porcelain stool, is far more effective for evacuating the bladder and bowels. With the left knee pressed up against the descending colon and the internal organs squeezed, elimination is encouraged. Sitting primly on the Western toilet, no pressure is applied nor action stimulated.

One consequence of this design difference is that those who use upright Western-style toilets are great consumers of laxatives. Poor elimination of waste and toxins from the body is a, if not the, major cause of illness and eventually, hospitalization. Your medical chart won't say, ―Brought down by being backed up,‖ but that's the truth.

I suspect you are tired of straining to produce some results, as well. My Abhyanga massage teacher, Dr. Nedungadi, liked to pantomime the constipated patient on the toilet…teeth and fists clenched, eyes bugging out of the head, deep grunting breaths and finally an exhausted, ―Thank you!‖ Few of us are totally unfamiliar with this tortured experience. If this is basically your bowel's story, you have the power to change it.

With straining can come bleeding and hemorrhoids, which are part of my old story.

HEMORRHOIDS, INACTIVITY, DIET AND WEIGHT

I think pregnancy is when I first noticed my bulging rectum, and during a prenatal examination the doctor confirmed I had already given birth to my first hemorrhoid. I was horrified, thinking _roids were limited to the domain of truck drivers and old, old people. How could this happen? I was 27!

Certainly, my added weight was putting pressure on my rectum. And I was less active, having gained close to 50 pounds before my delivery date. Even my feet spread out another half shoe size.

Looking back, I can see my pregnancy hemorrhoid was conceived by my overeating. In my head or not, I felt ravenously hungry for nine months. Having always been conscious of my weight, I had a great excuse for eating with abandon. Even if I watched my weight, my waist had disappeared, might as well have that second or even third serving of a sweet dessert.

Unaccustomed to the job I gave them, my intestines had trouble processing all the excess food and fats. YogaSir explains we store fat in the lower half of our body as it is the shortest trip, traveling from the large intestine or colon nearby to the hips, butt and belly. Moving fat cells all the way up to our backs and upper arms typically happens when we have exhausted the storage units in our lower trunk.

In its wisdom, the body works hard to store no fat around or near organs, to protect their proper functioning. Only when we've run out of hiding places for fat does it wrap around the heart, liver and other organs.

My pregnant self was eating way too many carbohydrates, probably eating for three and that means pooping for three. No wonder I felt the urge to push so hard.

TUMMY MUSCLES ARE IMPORTANT

As a pregnant woman, I couldn't activate my abdominal muscles properly. They were stretched to their maximum, and no longer even visible to me. Place your hands on the strong muscular wall below the naval and do Dr. Nedungadi's pantomime: push as if forcing a bowel movement. Can you feel those muscles contract, assisting the large intestine by giving a good squeeze?

Whenever I meet with someone who wants to change their bowels' performance, I look at the amount of belly fat they are carrying. When fat is really out of control, it is called an apron, hanging off the front of the body. I once sat next to a man on a plane with such a giant apron; he couldn't bring the tray table down for the flight attendant to place his meal. —Well,‖ I thought to myself, —Maybe he will wisely skip this meal.‖ But no, he placed the tray on his gut and inhaled every morsel.

I will bet my life savings though, that tasting was the only pleasant part of his eating experience. Digestion was clearly going to be painful for his overworked system, weighed down by stored fat. And with such a weak apron, he would have little assistance pushing out the remains of the meal. Ugh. Having already bet my life savings, I will have to bet my next life's savings that he has a bleeding anus, as well, as he struggles unnaturally to accomplish one of our most natural acts.

So how hard can we push, anyway? What is the right amount of pressure, to avoid hemorrhoids and straining?

In general, a good rule to follow is to not exert any harder than you would blowing your nose while seated on the toilet. In fact, as a way of retraining yourself to comfortably pass solids, you can sit on the toilet and consciously blow your nose, getting familiar with that level of pressure on the bowels.

But learning about pushing is merely an interim step in this new relationship you are creating with your elimination system. When everything is working in top form, there is little or no pushing. Solids exit the body as painlessly as when the food entered.

Make Energy, Not Cement

I've yet to meet an overeater who pigs out on vegetables or fruits. When we overeat, it is usually succumbing to cravings for bulk, for carbohydrates, the Comfort Foods. In the West, it is typically wheat. In the East, rice is the drug of choice. In both places, excess fat and sugar accompany these primary starches.

Living in both places, I acclimate to the overeating of the culture! Whether consuming too many cookies or toast bread, I turn my digestive system into a cement mixer.

The cement mixer metaphor works well for me. I imagine slowly grinding dry sand and stone with water, cranking hard to wet the heavy mass and move it on and out.

When I'm eating well, I have quite a speedy gut. Within eight hours of eating I usually see a meal exit. But on those days when I have eaten more than three servings of wheat or other starches, show time is delayed indefinitely.

The secret to consuming food that becomes energy and not cement is about what you decide to eat; or more accurately, who is making the decision.

When I get in trouble on the toilet, it is because Mr. Tongue picked the menu.

I think that proverb is so wise, I'm going to repeat it: When I get in trouble on the toilet, it is because Mr. Tongue picked the menu.

Mr. Tongue only has one criterion for admission: what does it taste like? He has no interest or involvement with the foreign matter once it leaves his domain. He has no idea about nutritional value, the ease of digestion or the difficulties facing the rectum. He is the Master of Impulse, both in speaking and eating. And when I allow Mr. Tongue to be impulsive, the rest of my life pays the price. As our grandmothers told us, —once on the lips, forever on the hips.‖ A saying, incidentally, that means nothing to Mr. Tongue.

Curiously, Mr. Tongue is the only muscle in the body attached at only one end. No wonder he needs restraint, in his speaking and eating.

As an interim step when rewriting the story of your bowels, it is wise to consult Miss Stomach about what you are planning to ingest. How much work will it be? What time of day are you asking her to remain open and active? Is she already full and busy?

WHAT ABOUT EATING MEAT

For years, I or members of my family flirted with partial or full-blown vegetarianism. Certain events triggered the change, like reading Upton Sinclair's The Jungle, about the horrors of the Chicago slaughterhouses in the 1920s.

I remember the only time my father sent me from the dinner table to my room, without finishing my meal, was when I sang, —When lips meet lips‖ as I was putting a hot dog in my mouth. He considered my behavior an insult to the cook, my mother. I never intended to hurt my mother; I was insulting the hot dog manufacturer.

Our digestive and elimination systems are those of an herbivore, that is, a non meat-eating creature. We aren't designed to digest meat, so no wonder it is such hard work for our bodies. Meat is complex muscle mass, it takes a lot of gastric juice and peristalsis to break it down and move the unusable out of the body.

Dr. Nedungadi asked two questions that made vegetarians out of most of my massage class. —Why do you want to make your large intestine an animal burial ground?‖ and —Why do you want to ingest the fear the animal felt at the time of slaughter?‖ I invite you to answer these questions for yourself. The good doctor also would ask us if we wanted to be able to accurately guess, —Who are your students who eat beef?‖

Of course!

—Just look for the ones who walk like the cow, he said, demonstrating with a slow bent over gait, his posterior sticking out.

Yogis stress the importance of eating live food. Swami Rama asked his disciples to throw a piece of meat and some grain or seeds on the ground and see which one grows. His students learned that meat is dead and lacks any life force.

Not only are we not created to eat meat, we don't eat carnivores, either. Tigers, dogs and other meat eaters are not part of our diet.

Remember Elvis Presley's death and autopsy? Found dead on his toilet, silk pajama bottoms at his feet. Was Elvis pushing so hard that he passed a clot to his brain? The coroner revealed Elvis had five pounds of undigested meat in his colon.

My first Ayurvedic massage, at the Birla Center for Hast Jyotish in Cheneville, Quebec, Chandan, my masseur, said to me, —You don't eat meat, do you?

Was he psychic? —How do you know? I asked.

Doing reflexology, he was squeezing the part of my left foot that represented the descending colon. —Your colon is so soft, no hard spots, he explained.

Years later, after completing my own studies in Ayurveda and reflexology, a massage client called me from her hospital bed.

—Bethany, I had half of my stomach removed five days ago, and I haven't been able to move my bowels. I am in agony, but they won't give me anything, for fear of bursting my stitches. Can you help me?

I asked Emma to put her nurse on the phone. —They aren't comfortable with that kind of care, she whispered. Instead, I told Emma and she told a visiting friend about the spot on the left foot, the magic button that Chandan had first shown me. —Work in a clockwise fashion, press hard and keep circling down and around, you'll get the bowels moving, I instructed.

Less than 10 minutes later, my phone rang again. A jubilant Emma on the line, —It worked! The nurses can't believe it! I feel so good, Bethany! Sharing the joy we experience when nature takes her course, I said to Emma, —I'm so happy for you. I do hope you named it after me!" We laughed together, as I have with other clients, who shared their painful secret and changed the story of their bowels.

During our Abhyanga massage course, Dr. Nedungadi taught us about what he called the, —Million dollar button." Located at the cleft of the chin, it is linked to the bowel meridian, one of many invisible lines on the body that run from top to toe. Dr. Nedungadi showed us how to help a constipated client by simply massaging this button. He also encouraged us when our own system got backed up to sit and squeeze the chin cleft, appearing to be deep in thought, but more accurately, deep in hope!

NO MEAT, LITTLE WHEAT, LESS SWEET

Beyond meat and wheat, the bowels struggle with sweets. Of course, the bowels aren't alone in being overwhelmed with our sugary diet. The poor pancreas forever has to fire up at different times of day and night to ramp our insulin factory up and down.

My own awakening to the incompatibility of sweets with my process of elimination came in India. I was enjoying a 12-day cleanse, consuming only limejuice with a taste of jaggery (natural brown sugar) and a pinch of cayenne pepper. This drink helps the body detox and purify; the lime cleanses, the sugar (maple syrup is great) provides some energy and the pepper keeps the Pitta digestive fires burning. *Only do this cleanse under doctor's supervision. Certain body types (particularly Pitta Dosha) can develop bleeding ulcers.*

During the fast, I was also doing three hours or more of Yoga a day, including breathing exercises, which included rectum locks.

Taking a drive with a neighbor on Day 10 of the fasting cleanse, we stopped in a busy marketplace to do an errand. I sat in the air-conditioned car and absent-mindedly read the store signs. —Amul Ice Cream" one screamed at me, in bright colors.

I instantly became aware of Mr. Tongue actually pulsing. I was stunned by the sensation, as I had honestly not missed any food at all during the cleanse. Before I could mentally translate the sensation into a thought, I felt my rectum squeeze tightly, uttering a clear, —no!"

King Rectum is the real author of my bowel's story. In that moment, sitting in the back seat of an SUV in Bangalore, I ended a chronic health problem. For decades, I have had an itchy rectum. Rarely have I gotten my courage up to talk with anyone about it, so forbidden are such below the belt conversations. With or without hemorrhoids (yes, I had that banding procedure done…what a way to blow $5000!) I periodically have such a terrific desire to scratch my anus, it has been awful. One health practitioner theorized I wasn't being careful in my wiping, so I became scrupulous in this process, even buying a commercial disposable, medicated wipe for a squeaky clean anus. But nothing stopped the itching.

King Rectum stopped it, telling me clearly that ice cream was no longer on the menu. By restricting my sugar intake, I ended the itch at the end.

TRAINING YOUR LITTLE PONY

Somewhere along my own path of rewriting my bowel's story, I came to think of my whole system of elimination as a pet pony. This pony required my attention, my disciplined training, my daily repetitive instruction. I committed myself to having perfectly functioning bowels, bowels that produced a movement every morning within five to 15 minutes of arising from bed.

Dr. Nedungadi advised a healthy being spends the night *parallel* to the earth, wakes and becomes *perpendicular*, and then sits up to *poop*. That simple. That easy. That natural. The Three Ps.

I found my bowels were particularly unreliable when I traveled. Thinking of the pony, I realized she was unfamiliar with a new barn, a new ring to walk around in, different food and water. No wonder she didn't perform on schedule. I needed to be especially attentive to her new surroundings; I needed to accommodate this change.

Long believing that my mind and body are not two but one, I work on the physical, mental and emotional levels when addressing a health problem.

I knew that my best bowel movements were at home, in the privacy of my own bathroom. (By the way, ladies, I don't advise having sex with any man that you can't comfortably have a bowel movement around. There is something Not Right about allowing intimacy on one level and being unable to relax in another normal natural act with the same person present. Consult your bowels about what you want to eat, as well as whom you sleep with!)

When traveling, I can't bring my bathroom with me, but I do bring my routine. Here is my 10-point plan for Good Bowel Health. Start with these steps, you can modify anything later.

1. Know what to avoid: no meat, less wheat, little sweet. Limit wheat to one serving per day, you can add more as bowels regulate.
2. Know the side effects of medications you take: can they cause sluggishness or constipation?
3. Know whom to consult: King Rectum and Miss Stomach; Mr. Tongue is of little help, except when it comes to poison!
4. Make sure green, yellow or red vegetables are the largest serving on your noon and evening plate. Veggies provide the fiber for a clean sweep of the bowels.
5. Always begin the day with fruit. A green smoothie is super. For best results in cold weather, eat a bowl of old fashioned oats for breakfast. Bonus: oats lower cholesterol, pulling fats out of the body.
6. Eat the big meal of the day in the middle of the day.
7. Eat very light at night, little starch, nothing after 6 p.m., and avoid eating cold and hot foods at the same time.
8. Snack on raw vegetables, fresh fruit, nuts and light foods. Sniff essential oils for a special no-calorie treat.
9. Drink eight glasses of room-temperature water or herbal tea daily.
10. Go to the toilet expecting a bowel movement at the same time every day. Sit for a while, relaxed. If you want to read, do so. Don't push harder than blowing your nose pressure. If nothing happens, don't judge yourself. Be patient, you have a lot of letting go to do.

In Ayurvedic medicine, we are advised that ideally, one should have as many poops as meals each day. Further, we are cautioned to not eat a meal unless you have evacuated your bowels since the last meal, that is, don't eat on top of an undigested meal. My daily elimination is typically two movements and what a friend calls, —the bonus.‖

Our systems are not all identical, given our *Doshas*. Pay attention to when you naturally find yourself having a movement. I am a morning pooper. I am aware of this, and therefore I treat my pony accordingly.

After I rise, I drink plenty of water, up to 16 ounces; to replenish the water my body has lost during the night, by sweating, digestion and other body functions.

I recommend room or body temperature water, as it is easiest for the body to process. Warmth encourages the bowels; it helps move the action along.

More than 50 years ago, one of the pioneers in the US fitness movement, Bonnie Prudden, (www.bonnieprudden.com) began instructing her students on a fail safe way to drink eight glasses of water a day. Stack eight coins on one end of the counter or windowsill by the kitchen sink. Every time a glass of water is consumed, move a coin to the other side of the counter or sill. At the end of the day, it is easy to check to make sure all eight coins traveled, or its time to drink more water.

I recall hearing how Rena Marcotte, founder and operator of Maple Lane Nursing Home in Barton, Vermont, toileted her patients. Rena's son Gary tells the story of the early days of the facility, when his mother single- handedly cared for 14 patients. —I remember she would bring a glass of prune juice to every resident each morning,‖ Gary said. —Then she would come around again with a cup of hot coffee for everyone.‖

—The third time she came around, she put them each on the toilet. It worked every time.‖ Rena was a master trainer of ponies.

For the 11 nights and 12 days in silence at the Vipassana Meditation Course, 20 women shared a common bathroom. I had no control over the menu or meal times and only about 20 minutes every day to walk. We were asked to not practice Yoga or any other form of exercise, but to keep ourselves focused for the 10 hours of daily meditation.

I told my pony before we left that I would be gentle and do whatever I could to keep our routine. Each morning, I rose and drank my water. I then squatted into the posture I do to encourage a movement, the very same position used for the Indian style toilet. This squat activates the descending colon, as the left knee and thigh are pushing against the colon, encouraging movement downwards. Lift the left heel off the floor to put more pressure on the area.

During the first two hours of seated meditation each day I periodically pulsed and locked my rectum. On the fourth morning at the course, immediately following the two-hour morning meditation, I had a movement.

A light breakfast was served, where I restricted myself to fruit and hot milk only. Most days I would also have a cup of hot water. As a yogi, I do not drink caffeine and limit alcohol.

Following this first meal of the day, I would take a 20-minute walk, which was typically followed by a second bowel movement.

I followed this routine for my entire stay at the Vipassana center, and it never varied. When I think of all the hours I sat on a concrete floor, which is one way of encouraging the production of hemorrhoids, I was so pleased with my pony. I feel the rectum locking had a lot to do with prevention of _roid development, as this is my weakness.

At mid day, I ate a large meal of vegetables and rice. At 5 I had warm milk and fruit again. I did not expect the bonus until the following day, and my pony complied.

No matter where I am, I believe it is wisest to not eat much at night, and certainly not after 6 p.m.

I can hear lots of readers slamming the book shut with these dinner instructions, or at least beginning their power whines, —That just won't work for me, that is impossible.‖ After all, many folks don't have dinner until 9 p.m. or later.

Well, enjoy your irregularity is all I can say. Unless you have a very cooperative system, at least in the early days of training your pony, late night eating must be avoided. Eating after dark makes your stomach work hard all night. Many clients will say, —But I get so hungry after 9 or 10.‖ Ayurveda and Yoga again explain that we mistake the activation of the natural evening digestive cycle as a message of hunger. In actuality, the body is just firing up to do some digesting of the current stomach contents. The sensation you feel is not hunger, your body is not calling for more food.

However, if you put more food in late at night, you will never burn the stored fat. Your body will be too busy dealing with your full tummy.

RAMPING UP YOUR CAMPAIGN

For those of us who are Type A personalities, even when it comes to wanting to have award winning bowel stories, yes you can jumpstart the process and get your pony moving.

Constipation is not an isolated aspect of your life. Rather, it is another one of those flashing lights on your body's dashboard, reminding you to —check engine.‖

In this case, check engine requires you do a thorough review of your lifestyle and habits.

To generalize, in my practice I have found that constipation is closely linked to one or more of the following challenges:

- Being anxious
- Fear of someone close, like spouse, roommate or parent
- Perfectionism
- Being a pleaser
- Being more outer than inner focused
- Hoarding, collecting, over-acquiring
- Being inactive and inert

BEING ANXIOUS, FEARFUL

When we have difficulty relaxing, our bowels share that problem. Being uptight (the slang is —being a tight ass‖) our bowels, particularly our rectum, don't fully open and release. When tension is great in the body, that fecal matter can remain impacted for days and days.

In the early 1990s, I spent a summer at Duke University's Divinity School, as part of the local pastor training program of the United Methodist Church. I was randomly assigned a female roommate to share campus housing. My roommate, Mitzy, was a southern woman, and our differences were quickly apparent. I'm sure she regarded me as too open, informal and perhaps even ill-mannered.

I immediately had trouble having a bowel movement. In those days, I knew little about tending my system of elimination, other than to have a packet of matches in the bathroom to camouflage any odors I might leave behind.

Mitzy was orderly and organized. Before we sat to eat, she would wash the food preparation items and fill the sink with hot water. Her bedroom was full of neatly folded items and her study desk was carefully organized. Truly there was method in her Methodism. I quickly began to feel inadequate, aware of her glances at my desk, my bed, my dresser top.

My bowels also noted the tension of our arrangement and decided to shut down completely. A few frantic calls to my husband sent me shopping for my first container of an orange flavored natural laxative drink. Four days of this drink left my belly incredibly distended and gassy, but no other action occurred in the southern hemisphere. My evening calls back home were tense and terse. —That stuff is not working! I would whisper accusatively, as if he was somehow remote-controlling my bowels. He kept reassuring me and saying it would work.

A dirigible in bed at night, I would wake to sounds of my own flatulence, and Mitzy's crisp, annoyed voice, —Was that you? from the adjoining bedroom. Oh man, yeah, I guess so.

I spent long sessions in the toilet, but noxious tooting was all I could achieve. After one such lackluster performance, I returned to the breakfast table. —I need to ask if you are smoking marijuana in the bathroom, Mitzy said, with all the tact of a warden in a women's prison.

I was shocked. —I don't smoke marijuana, I don't smoke anything! I said, wondering what kind of pastor she thought I was, or she was.

—Well, what are you doing with those matches in the bathroom, and spending so much time in there?"

I wanted to scream, —Trying to have a dump that won't come because you make me so nervous!" Instead, I muttered something about a poor man's air freshener and went to class.

After close to a week, on a lovely sunny afternoon between classes, I found an isolated bathroom on the divinity school campus and let go and let God. I vowed that I would no longer let Mitzy run me or my bowels.

Perhaps you have a similar source of discomfort in your environment that makes your bowels withdraw. Use your constipation as you use any flashing light on the dash: notice what you need to change.

PERFECTIONIST, PLEASER, OUTER FOCUSED

When we are dependent on the opinions of others for our self-confidence and identity, we often have little awareness of our bodies or moods. We are tuned to The Other, how to please them, engage them, receive their praise. Rather than being the star in our own life, we play the part of best supporting actress in the lives of Others.

Appearances become overly important when we have this mindset, and we can devote hours to makeup, hair and clothing in the morning, leaving little or no time for such a private act as a bowel movement. Whether we make time for a movement or not does not matter to others, yet we are living for their approval!

Like my experience as the fearful, tense divinity student, you may find your bowels don't seem connected to you, and refuse to cooperate. You don't make time to sit quietly on the toilet, as you don't like time alone of any kind. Perhaps you see time spent alone as being taken from The Other, who might well be waiting for you to prepare breakfast, pack a bag lunch or drop them off at school. One's own bowel movement is an after-thought at the most, and this is a metaphor for one's whole life. When we don't put ourselves first, our bowels tell that story. They end up needing to be emptied at the most inopportune times, because we have ignored them for hours. Suddenly, we can delay no longer and an emergency strikes.

We must learn to relax and provide ourselves the necessary attention and self care to be healthy, functioning human beings. Earlier, I mentioned the family member who inevitably needs to have a movement when on her weekly grocery shopping trip. Shopping, she is relaxed and not totally focused on serving others. She moves at a more leisurely pace through the store, allowing her whole body to release tension and unwind. In this state of calm and inner peace, her bowels signal naturally to her that they are ready to empty. And when she is ready to pay more attention to herself, her bowels will give her a natural, daily signal, right at home, in the privacy of her own, clean, personal bathroom.

HOARDING, COLLECTING, OVER-ACQUIRING

The brilliant metaphysical pioneer Louise Hay first awakened me to the connection between not letting go of things and constipation. In her classic guide (a must for all family libraries) <u>Heal Your Body A to Z, the Mental Causes for Physical Illness and the Metaphysical Way to Overcome Them</u> Hay describes her understanding of constipation.

—If you came to me as a client with a problem of constipation, I would know you had some sort of belief in limitation and lack and therefore, were mentally frightened to let go of anything out of fear of not being able to replace it. It could also mean you were holding onto an old painful memory of the past and would not let go. You might have a fear of letting go of relationships that no longer nourish you, or a job that is unfulfilling, or some possessions that are now unusable. You might even be stingy about money. Your dis-ease would give me many clues to your mental attitude.

Hay helps such individuals learn the principle of releasing and letting go, of learning to trust the natural flow of life that they need not cling and fear they won't be provided for. Further, she often encourages them to begin to clean out closets, junk drawers and spare rooms, letting go of all that isn't serving them. Giving away useless things and making way for the new, Hay says constipation often takes care of itself.

In this spirit, I also recommend that, as part of the 10-point plan; those serious about changing their Bowel's Story begin to lighten their load of stuff and activities. Letting go of clothes, shoes and household items you haven't touched in several years is very freeing. Letting go of relationships or pastimes that no longer feed you or leave you feeling good about yourself is another important step. If in doubt, throw it out!

Incorporating a weekly day of fasting into your life is another powerful way to break your pattern of craving and clinging. When we fast, we become immediately aware of how much time we spend thinking about food. First, we plan to shop and make sure we have the funds to purchase the food. We shop, carrying it to and from the store into the car and house. We put it away, only later to take it out and prepare it. We dispose of the recyclables and garbage. We eat the meal. We digest the meal. We wait to eliminate the meal.

On a fast day, all of that time is freed up for something else. You notice food may well consume more of your time than is necessary. If you have become someone who lives to eat, rather than eats to live, a weekly fast is a wonderful step toward ending this bondage.

On Day One, have your evening meal, don't eat at all on Day Two the following day, and break the fast with breakfast (now you know the meaning of the word) on Day Three. Beyond the mental clarity and lessons this practice allows, you will also give your digestive and eliminative systems a nice rest.

Whatever actions you are willing to take, make sure you make the mental link between emptying your life of the old and awakening your bowels to a natural pattern of regularity. When you're stuck, you're stuck.

INACTIVE AND INERT

We refer to it as a bowel movement for a reason. Your body actively works hard from the moment you put food into your body to wring all the nutritional value out of it and then send it packing.

By remaining physically active, we can greatly assist in this process of digestion and elimination. Yoga poses that involve twisting and bending over are especially encouraging to the bowel. Make sure you are honest with yourself when assessing your activity level. I have a friend who tried countless methods of ending her constipation, with very limited success. Only when she took a walking tour of France did she find her bowels began to function as designed. She needed to get moving to have a movement.

I have known people, so desperate to get unplugged, they have worn a very tight waist or cinched a tight belt and caused great discomfort and their bowels roared. No one wants to take such painful measures to achieve something so natural.

A WELL-TUNED BOWEL

When our bowels are working, they are busy and productive. What goes in must come out. Still, remember that the majority of waste your body excretes leaves on your exhale, in the form of a gas. Some researchers claim upward of 70 percent of the elimination our body casts off occurs through breathing. Only the solids and liquids rely on the bowel and bladder.

When I first started to study the anatomy, I had my doctor husband draw my organs with a marker on my skin. I wanted to know where parts and pieces of the system were, and where it might be blocked. Right off, I found it neat to learn that, like the *chakras,* my digestive and elimination systems work in a clockwise fashion. That means just by rubbing your stomach down your left side, across, up the right and across the top encourages healthy movement. I often encourage constipated individuals to sit on the toilet and rub their bellies, clockwise. The comforting warmth of the hand is frequently enough to get the party started.

Right below your ribcage is the transverse colon, bringing the food that has come up from the right side of the body across the front and heading down to the descending colon, on the left side of the body. Now you understand my earlier reference to rubbing the bottom left lower side of the left foot, as it simulates where the descending colon actually lies.

In the stomach, the food is broken down into manageable consistency and passed to the small intestine, where the majority of nutritional absorption occurs. From the small intestine, the roughage and other byproducts of little value are pushed along into the large intestine. Within the large intestine and headed to the descending colon, some final nutrients are extracted and the fats are pulled out and absorbed by the body. If you place your left hand low, tucked up against the left edge of your belly, you are near the end of your meal's journey, where the descending colon is heading for the rectum. Basically, this lower left side is where, God willing, Elvis will leave the building.

My dear friend, the late Florence Alice Coburn, who I had the honor of serving as a guardian for the last 12 years of her life, had to learn all about her sphincter and its magical abilities after she turned 60 years of age.

Raised in mental institutions, Florence never enjoyed the luxury of tuning into her body. She was told by the facility staff, with all of the others in her ward, when it was time to pee and poop. A bank of toilets lined the wall of the bathroom, with no walls between them for privacy. Dutifully trained by outsiders, Florence would walk to the bathroom with the other patients on the ward, as ordered, and have a bowel movement. Not unlike my little dogs' performances, when they are sent outside to do their duty.

Hospital bowel training was created for the convenience of the staff. When Florence decided she wanted to leave the mental hospital, she faced many social challenges. One of her greatest struggles was around the absence of self-directed toileting skills. Living in her apartment after a lifetime of dormitory-style living, when Florence got frustrated, she would spread her legs and urinate, acting out the original meaning of —pissed off.‖

Getting to know her bowels and their function was difficult, as she had never learned that the tiny pulsing signal emitted by her sphincter meant, —The bowel needs to be emptied.‖ The anal sphincter is a circular muscle that closes and opens the anus. Learning to decipher this simple yet vital message as a senior citizen was tough, but Florence persevered. She also had the unusual problem of being unable to poop when alone, radically opposite from the need for privacy most of us have. In time, Florence was proudly announcing, —I decided to go poop,‖ and headed for the bathroom to move her bowels. A real rite of passage in her emancipation.

CHAPTER 9

CHAIR YOGA AND COMMON AILMENTS

Not only does Yoga provide the most practical approach to attaining a high level of physical fitness, but it stabilizes the emotions and elevates one's mental attitude.

Richard Hittleman

We all know the dangerous cycle: we feel stiff and achy, so we avoid exercise, only to feel stiffer and achier. As children, we were cautioned not to crack our knuckles, as we would cause arthritis.

Yoga blows the roof off these myths about the value of inactivity. Being gentle with ourselves and listening to our bodies, we inch up toward pain, but stop before we get there. When you live as if your body is your best friend, you treat yourself kindly.

Tight, tense joints are desperately hungry for the magical lubricant, synovial fluid. Yet, ironically, it is only released when the joint moves. So, if we choose to consciously sit as inert and frozen as we can while watching television, our stiff joints receive no oil! But if we regularly flex and move and rotate and bend our joints as they are designed, synovial fluid will flood them with comfort.

And as for cracking our knuckles?

—The unmistakable sound of a knuckle cracking is caused by a bubble or gas cavity in the synovial fluid, forming between finger joints,‖ according to Dr. Greg Kawchuk, a professor of rehabilitation at the University of Alberta, and lead author of the 2014 synovial bubble study.

Releasing tension and pain, alleviating aches and anxiety, and improved thinking come with the territory in the Land of Yoga.

Stimulating the brain with increased oxygen and new ways of perceiving, Yoga's value goes beyond the physical and spiritual. Every time we try a new yoga pose or breath a unique 60,000 mile network of neurons gets activated. With each new thought and movement, neuro-connections extend and intertwine. Changing constantly, the brainpower is forever growing, toward higher states of consciousness.

Thousands and thousands of years of experience with this proven life giving technique are reaffirmed daily by Yoga practitioners around the world. Unless otherwise stated, Chair Yoga is done once or twice a day, on an empty stomach, seated, before the noon and evening meals.

YOGA TAKES ON THE SKIN ULCER

An overweight woman, Rose, over the age of 65, had a painful skin ulcer on her left shin for many years. Open and raw, it was about 8 inches long and 4 to 5 inches wide; the patch was dark black in the center, circled by an angry red section. The whole area hurt, and it burned in the center.

Because of her weight and bad knees (bad knees are a direct result of being overweight) Rose was limited to doing her yoga breathing and poses while seated.

Rose's Daily Program

Three locks: Exhale fully, swallow and lock neck (tucking chin deeply into chest), suck naval back to spine and hold, pull rectum up and hold. Hold until you need to breathe. Inhale, tip head back then forward, exhale, swallow, lock and hold. Prevents health problems, especially in throat and systems of digestion and elimination.

Toe to Top Seated Light Warm Ups

At the beginning of her second month of doing Chair Yoga daily, Rose showed YogaSir the patch of irritated skin: what had been red was now the normal color of her flesh and the dark black center was turning red. The ulcerous wound was drying up and closing.

YOGA, SELF CONFIDENCE AND FLEXIBILITY

Susan is married, a working mother of two, in her mid 40s. She and her husband own and operate two booming enterprises that require lots of their time and attention. Feeling exhausted and stuck, Susan decided to meditate to overcome her pattern of worrying. She also expressed a desire to gain more confidence and move forward in her life. Chronically constipated and very stiff from a lack of any exercise, she knew she wanted to loosen up and lose about 20 pounds. On many levels, Susan was holding on, clinging and clutching to the old.

Susan's Daily Program

All 10 breathing exercises listed in the Chapter 5 sample routine.
Toe to Top Light Warm Ups

Seated Forward Bend: In chair, extend legs out in front of you and reach out to touch toes, dropping forehead toward knees. Hang and breathe. Repeat three-five times.

Seated Rag Doll: Sit. While inhaling, raise arms above head with limp wrists. Swing down to the floor with a forced exhale, even adding a grunt or sound from deep in the belly like —ha‖ to fully empty lungs. . If hands touch floor, bring them back behind feet as far as possible. Hang loose with head in lap. Repeat up to five times.

Early in her practice, Susan would seem surprised she couldn't touch her toes or bend in a certain direction. —This won't move,‖ she would say, pointing to a part of her body. During other sessions, she referred to herself as —it.‖ Such references are a classic example of the disconnected relationship we can have with our bodies, a connection Yoga reconnects.

After one month of Yoga, Susan got her hair streaked, announcing it is something she had wanted to do for years, but lacked confidence. She added daily walks to her morning routine. She further reported a loss of three inches around her waistline and shrieked with joy the day she could almost touch her toes. —I love Yoga! I can't wait to see more changes in me.‖

In her second month, she touched her toes for the first time in memory. —I couldn't even do this as a teenager!‖ she beamed.

Focusing on her constipation, she slowly realized she needed three conditions to have regular movements: privacy, time and something to read at her side. With this newfound awareness, Susan began —training her pony‖ in a daily pattern of elimination.

YOGA IMPROVES EYESIGHT

Sherrie came to Yoga for overall relaxation, reducing aches and pains and a general desire to stave off signs of advancing age.

She never considered Yoga would improve her eyesight. But Clock Face produced an unexpected gift for Sherrie.

—I went for my annual eye exam and my doctor asked, _What have you been doing? Your eyes have improved.'‖ Sherrie told him about Clock Face, a practice her teacher said would help round her eyeballs, which were naturally getting flat with age.

Sherrie's Daily Program

Toe to Top Light Warm Ups

Clock Face: Imagine your face is a clock. Think of random hours, and look at the appropriate area of your face. For example, three o'clock is directly to your right, and 12 is straight up. Move only your eyes. Go in both directions, diagonally and other ways. Breathe slowly and deeply. Strengthens eyes and restores roundness to eyeball. Preferable to do with eyes open.

STIFFNESS FROM WHIPLASH DISAPPEARS

Patty is an active woman in her fifties, running a large family business that produces packaged foods. While she gets plenty of exercise on a daily basis, she also experienced plenty of aches and pains.

She came to Yoga because of problems with her joints, specifically her hips and neck. Like many people with chronic pain, she had decided she was just going to have to live with it. Beyond the normal wear and tear of aging, Patty's pain was related to an old whiplash injury.

Patty's Daily Program

Half Butterfly: Bring right foot up and place on left thigh, as close to hip as able. Sit like this as long as comfortable, working at your desk or watching television. With right hand, lift right knee up and push back down to further stimulate the hip and release the synovial fluid lubricant (simulates one butterfly wing flapping). Lift left heel off floor to increase the stretch. When ready, switch legs and repeat. Do often throughout the day. Finish with a nice full extension of each leg.

Rock the Twins: Bring right foot up and place on opposite knee. Lift up right leg, cradling like a baby from knee to foot, and rock side-to-side, loosening up hip. Switch legs.

Hip Circles: Pull left leg up to chest and lace hands around knee. Imagine your left thighbone is a large wooden spoon, and your buttock is a pot of chili on the stove. Your intention is to stir just the bottom of the chili pot. Slowly and subtly stir the chili, circling clockwise and counterclockwise, a small-refined circle. If you notice your foot is circling, you aren't stirring the pot. Focus on the hip joint only. Switch legs, repeat on right side.

Neck Release: Close eyes. Sit upright, yet comfortable. Take a deep inhale and as you exhale, allow your hardworking neck to fall into your chest. Continue breathing, letting the neck hang. With every exhale allow gravity to help your neck release more tightness, as you simply hang. Inhale and bring head back to center, exhaling as you turn the head gently to the right. Breathe here for a few breaths. Inhale. On the exhale turn the head gently to the left. Again, breathe here for a few moments. Inhale back to center, drop the head again on the exhale, hang and breathe. At your own pace, begin a series of slow circles with the neck, allowing yourself to release tension as you roll the head around the front to the back. Reverse directions and always make sure you are breathing. Do a few rounds and enjoy the release.

Arm Cradle: Drape right arm overhead and touch left ear. Place left hand on left shoulder. Inhale fully, right up into the upper lobes of the lungs. On the exhale, gently let the head fall to the right, as both elbows drop down more toward the sides. All of your focus is on the space between the two hands…allow it to open and stretch. Stay here for a few breaths. Switch to the other side and repeat process.

After a few months of practice, Patty reported her joints definitely had benefited from Yoga.

—When I don't do Yoga for awhile, they begin to hurt again. Then when I do some stretches, all is better! I know I am more flexible generally than I was before, too,‖ she said, adding with a smile, —Yoga is wonderful for aging bodies.‖

Unlike strenuous aerobic exercise, which builds lactic acid in the muscles and can create great fatigue, Yoga is a physical science that relaxes and energizes, creating no lactic acid.

Among the most powerful poses are the Light Warm-ups, exercises designed to free up energy blockages in the joints and muscles. When the life force or *Prana* isn't moving easily and freely throughout the mind and body, problems can easily arise on the physical, mental, emotional and spiritual planes.

The Light Warm Ups are ideal for young and old yogis, whether experienced or new to the practice. Considered the basics or foundation for more demanding poses, these moves loosen up and address rheumatic, digestive and stamina limitations.

When practicing the Warm Ups, you can concentrate on one or more fields. For some, experiencing the posture and the associated physical feelings provides plenty of satisfaction. Other students will enjoy tying the poses to the breath, synchronizing the inhale and exhale with specific movements to actually fuel the posture.

A third option for focusing your attention when practicing the Warm Ups is to sense energy moving throughout the body. Sometimes a specific part of the body, like the face or hands, will start to tingle, awakening you to the revitalized flow of energy.

Regardless of where you place your attention, remember to relax and enjoy. Don't feel self conscious or worry about not being able to do something. Chair Yoga is fun and you can easily customize any of the Warm Ups to suit your situation. The order of your practice is important. Always begin with breathing exercises, follow with Toe to Top Light Seated Warm Ups, then poses.

TOE TO TOP SEATED LIGHT WARM UPS

Do each posture the equivalent of four breaths

Feet and ankle series: Seated comfortably, lift feet off floor; roll ankles in a circle, both directions.

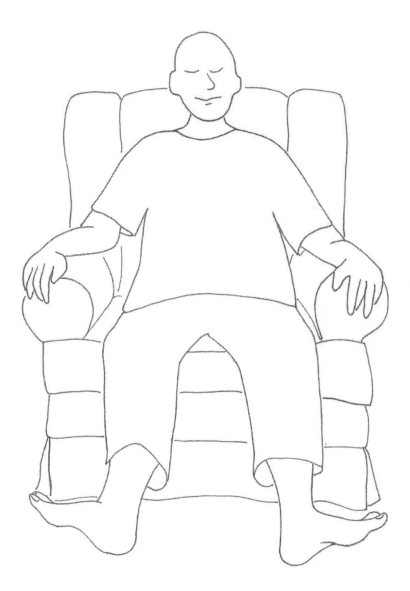

Place feet wide apart on floor and turn feet in and out, from pigeon-toed to duck-footed.

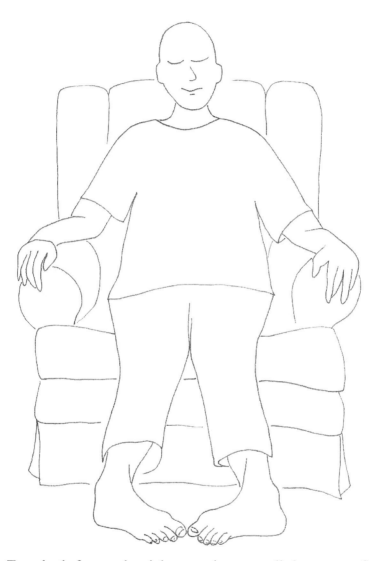

Turn both feet to the right, pressing toes all the way to floor. Go to the left and repeat.

Push pedals up and down, like the gas and brakes of a car, flexing feet as far back and then as far forward as possible. Make fists with the feet, then open and spread toes widely.

If in a class, wave at another foot in the room.

With feet on floor, scoop imaginary marbles or uncooked rice with feet, curling arches inward.

While sitting, stand on toes. Lift heels alternatingly, marching in place. March with feet flat on the floor, stimulating the whole body.

With feet flat on the floor, lift toes up only.

KNEES

Kneecap Contraction: stretch the legs out in front of you and support right leg with left underneath it. Inhale and retain the breath, tightening the muscles around the right knee, as if pulling the kneecap up toward the thigh. Hold for few counts, exhale and relax. Reverse sides and repeat with right leg underneath. Repeat five times on each leg.

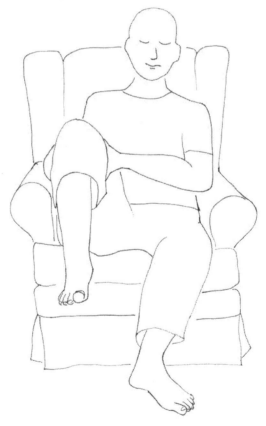

Knee Crank: Sit comfortably, pull left knee up and lace hands underneath the left thigh, in the crease of the knee, holding the weight of the thigh. Make circles with the lower leg, inhaling on the up swing and exhale on the down. Straighten the leg as much as able when foot heads toward ceiling. The rest of the body remains still! Circle 10 times in each direction and switch legs.

Massage knees, slow but strong. Use both hands on one knee, working all over and under to stimulate circulation. After massaging both knees with both hands, switch and place one hand on each knee for ongoing gentle massage. Massage both clockwise and counter-clockwise.

HIPS

Half Butterfly: Bring right foot up and place on left thigh, as close to hip as able. Sit like this as long as comfortable, working at your desk or watching television. With right hand, lift right knee up and push back down to further stimulate the hip and release the synovial fluid lubricant (simulates one butterfly wing flapping). Lift left heel off floor to increase the stretch. When ready, switch legs and repeat. Do often throughout the day. Finish with a nice full extension of each leg.

Rock the Twins: Bring right foot up and place on opposite knee. Lift up right leg, cradling like a baby from knee to foot, and rock side-to-side, loosening up hip. Switch legs.

Hip Circles: Pull left leg up to chest and lace hands around knee. Imagine your left thighbone is a large wooden spoon, and your buttock is a pot of chili on the stove. Your intention is to stir just the bottom of the chili pot. Slowly and subtly stir the chili, circling clockwise and counterclockwise, a small-refined circle.

If you notice your foot is circling, you aren't stirring the pot. Focus on the hip joint only. Switch legs, repeat on right side.

WAIST

Seated Twist: Sit upright. Reach right arm across chest, keeping it strong and straight. Continue reaching around, behind left shoulder. If able, hold back of chair, sliding hand along back of chair as far to right as possible. If on stool, reach around to grab right side of neck. Twist trims the waist and shoulders also benefit from this stretch. Keep fanny on seat. Turn head and look over right shoulder and continue to breathe. Take two complete breaths. Reverse, using left arm. Repeat up to five times on each side.

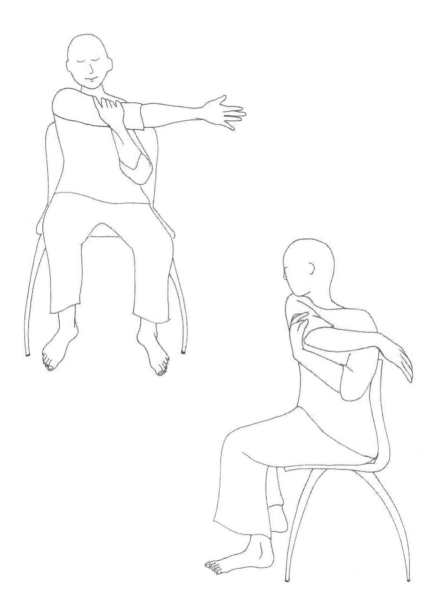

Seated Rag Doll: Sit. While inhaling, raise arms above head with limp wrists. Swing down to the floor with a forced exhale, even adding a grunt or sound from deep in the belly like —ha‖ to fully empty lungs. If hands touch floor, bring them back behind feet as far as possible. Hang loose with head in lap!

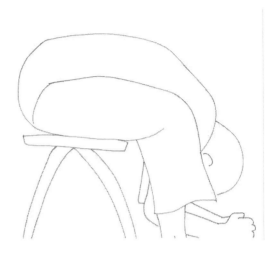

Repeat up to five times.

Carving a Waist: Inhale, lace and place hands behind head, arms open wide. Exhaling, touch right elbow to left knee. Inhaling as you come up, fall to the right side as low as possible. Inhale up. Exhaling, touch left elbow to right knee. Inhaling as you come up, fall to the left side as low as possible.

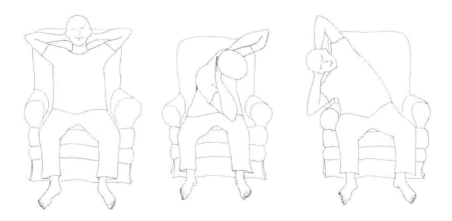

ELBOWS

Elbow Pumping: Sit, pump arms up and down, hands in fists. Activates heart and other organs, helps make blood.

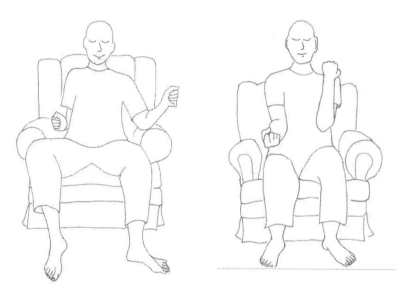

HANDS AND WRISTS

Halt: Put right arm straight out in front of you, with hand up, as if you are saying, —halt!‖ With other hand, pull fingertips back and release. Do three times. Then let right hand turn, so fingers are pointing downward and again, using left hand, pull fingers back, three times. Repeat on other side.

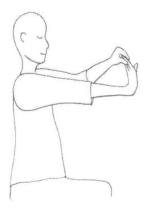 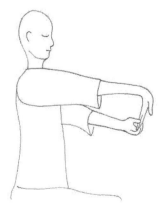

Hand Curl: Put both arms out in front and curl hands down and then flip hands back up so fingers are pointing upwards.

Wrist Rolls: sit with hands in fists, with hands together, thumbs touching, begin rolling fists in circles, keeping hands in contact with each other, as hands rise up in front of you and go over head, then reverse direction of roll and come back down. Do again and this time when overhead, split hands apart and have them roll down solo, with arms extended out to sides and back to lap.

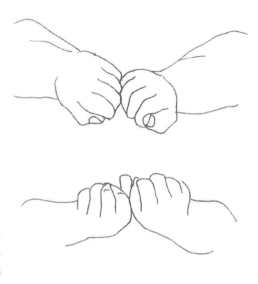

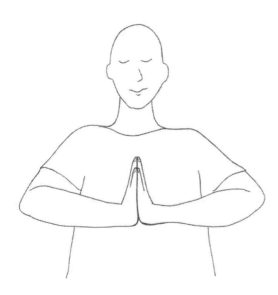

Pushing Prayer: put hands in prayer position, in front of chest, elbows straight out to sides. Using resistance, press hands and fingers against each other, keeping arms still. Do for two minutes.

Finger Push-ups: Open up left hand with palm facing right in front of you. Place right hand, finger tips only, on the tips of open left hand. Extend fingers flat so they touch each other, then pull back so only tips touch.

Repeat 20 times. Flip let hand so palm is facing up; repeat with right hand on top, sometimes known as —spider on the mirror‖! Do 20 times, flip left hand so it is on top with palm facing down and repeat.

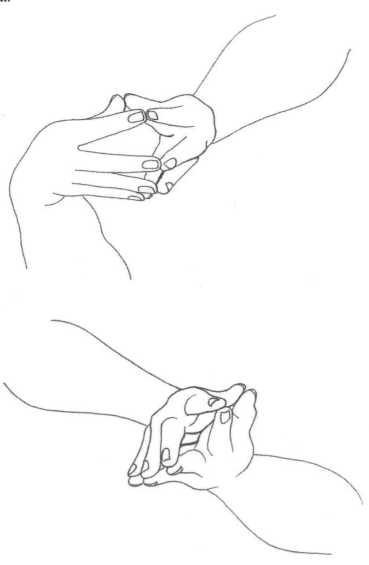

Fist and Flower: Inhale, clench fists tightly with thumb inside and hold breath, in the symbol of hostility. Exhale, open palms and fingers wide, in the symbol of hospitality. Repeat.

SHOULDERS AND NECK

Wing Circles: Close eyes. Place left hand on left shoulder, right hand on right shoulder. Circle your wings, work to bring elbows to touch each other in front. Reverse directions. Drop hands and circle shoulders in one direction and then the other, then circle the shoulders in opposite directions at the same time.

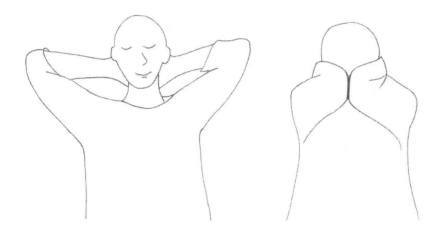

Open and Close Wings: Inhale, lace and place hands behind neck, opening arms out wide. On the exhale, squeeze arms together, trying to touch elbows and cover your face. Inhale and fully open wings. Repeat as long as it feels good.

Neck Release: Close eyes. Sit upright, yet comfortable. Take a deep inhale and as you exhale, allow your hardworking neck to fall into your chest. Continue breathing, letting the neck hang. With every exhale allow gravity to help your neck release more tightness, as you simply hang. Inhale and bring the head back to center, exhaling as you turn the head gently to the right. Breathe here for a few breaths. Inhale. On the exhale turn the head gently to the left. Again, breathe here for a few moments. Inhale back to center, drop the head again on the exhale, hang and breathe.

At your own pace, begin a series of slow circles with the neck, allowing yourself to release tension as you roll the head around the front to the back. Reverse directions and always make sure you are breathing. Do a few rounds and enjoy the release.

Psychic Union: Sit and close eyes. Lace hands behind back. Inhale deeply. When exhaling, fall forward, spine straight, bringing forehead as close to lap as possible, arms up behind you. Stay and breathe as long as comfortable. Relax into stretch, let gravity help you to fall even further down, lifting arms above you.

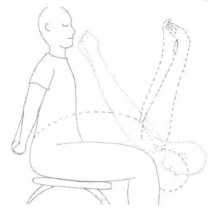

Locomotive: With hands in fists, and elbows bent, punch fists forward and then pull back, imitating the motion of connected train wheels. Reverse directions.

Arm Cradle: Drape right arm overhead and touch left ear. Place left hand on left shoulder. Inhale fully, right up into the upper lobes of the lungs. On the exhale, gently let the head fall to the right, as both elbows drop down more toward the sides. All of your focus is on the space between the two hands…allow it to open and stretch. Stay here for a few breaths. Switch to the other side and repeat process.

Vertical Handshake: Place right hand on center back, elbow is pointing upwards. Take left hand and bring behind back, reaching up toward right hand. Grasp shirt if needed (or have each hand hold the end of a towel, scarf or belt) and climb toward one another. See if you can shake hands. Upper elbow is ideally directly

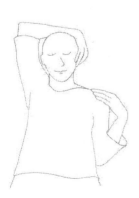
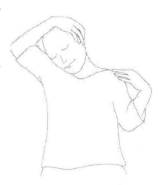

behind the head. For more of a challenge, look up. Reverse hands, placing left hand at top. Variation: Place right hand on center back. Take left hand and push right elbow down, stretching shoulder. Reverse hands.

Hand versus Head: Push right hand against side of head above ear, using resistance, inhaling through nose. Exhale. Place right hand at back of head, keep elbow out wide, inhale and push hand and head with resistance. Exhale. Repeat on other side of head with left hand. With palms close together, hold chin with thumb and forefinger and on the inhale push hands into chin and resist with chin pushing back. Repeat full series five times.

Circling Thumbs: With hands clasped together tightly keep thumbs up and circle arms around in front of you, quickly, following your thumbs with eyes. Circle in both directions.

FACE

Face: Sing out ―O‖ and ―Wee‖ with great enthusiasm, exaggerating the movement of the mouth! You're stretching it North to South and then East to West. Ahh…

Palming Forehead: with palms facing face, press heels of hands into forehead above brows, sliding all the way up to the hairline. Repeat, one hand pushing in and up, and then the other.

Rub Wrinkles Out: Cover face with warm hands, press face and pull hands away from nose out to ears, as if ironing or rubbing out wrinkles. Repeat.

ADD SUN SALUTE TO YOUR MORNING WARM UP!

The Sun Salutation is a classic warm up for a good day and a good Yoga class. Try this modified version of the morning salute, which does not require you get on the floor.

Rather than the floor, use a heavy chair, counter top, desk or table edge that won't budge.

Make sure you have plenty of room behind you. Face your counter edge or back of the chair, standing just close enough to touch.

1. Inhale, raise hands overhead, stretching backwards as far as comfortable.

2. Exhale, bring hands to prayer position at chest.

3. Inhale, raise hands overhead, stretching backwards as far as comfortable.

4. Exhale, bend forward and grasp back of chair or furniture edge.

5. Holding on, lean down with head the same height as arms and shoulders, stepping back as far as comfortable. Enjoy a few breaths.

6. Still holding on, exhale and lower head, shoulders, chest and belly while body is extended. Inhale, arch spine up, then drop back down again on exhale.

7. Still holding on, inhale, raise chin up and tip head back, puffing out chest.

8. Exhale, let go of chair, stand up slowly. Let arms and head hang down.

9. Inhale, raise hands overhead, stretching backwards as far as comfortable.

10. Exhale, bring hands to prayer position at chest.

Start with two Sun Salutations and build up to 10 or more. As your practice becomes stronger, challenge yourself by lowering the stretch. Use the seat of the heavy chair (or a low sturdy chest or coffee table) repeating the 10 steps at a lower height. *(My thanks to Bread and Puppeteer Elka Schumann for urging me to teach a modified Sun Salutation.)*

ALPHABETICAL LISTING OF COMMON AILMENTS AND CHAIR YOGA RESPONSE

ADDICTIONS:

Addictions to stimulants, cigarettes, sex, work, gambling, extreme sports, and other cravings

Even judges are ordering convicted lawbreakers with addiction problems to try a Yoga class. In a Texas courtroom, Judge Larry Standley sentenced James Lee Cross, struggling with substance abuse, to enroll in Yoga to get help managing his anger, after hitting his wife on New Year's Eve.

As you inhale, see this act as your grasping and grabbing, your expression of addiction. As you exhale, see the natural release of this habit of clinging. Experience the moment between inhalation and exhalation, feel the natural state of completeness, of having everything you need, of peace. All breathing exercises are useful. Smokers will especially find satisfaction with deep inhales and exhales.

Alternate Nostril Breathing: Hold right hand up to nose, with elbow slightly tucked to your side and shoulder relaxed. Left hand resting on thigh. Gently close right nostril with right thumb and inhale from the left. Close left nostril with ring finger and exhale from right. Keep left nostril closed and inhale from right. Close right nostril with thumb and exhale from left. These steps comprise one round. Retention of breath can be added between each inhale and exhale, to promote the development of muscle mass.

Rolled Pipe Tongue Cooling Breath: Roll tongue like a pipe, stick out of mouth and inhale, drawing air over tongue. If you can't roll your tongue, this is actually an inherited talent, do the *Hissing Breath*: Slightly open mouth, with teeth slightly parted and tongue planted behind lower teeth and inhale. For both styles of cooling breath, after inhaling, swallow and exhale through left nostril, holding right nostril closed with right thumb. Repeat five-eight times.

Furnace Breath: Inhale making soft snoring noise in throat, like a baby sleeping. Swallow to hold breath. Exhale from left nostril only, holding right closed with right thumb. Do eight complete cycles. Removes phlegm from the throat and improves digestion.

Diving: Sit upright, suck in stomach and hold it in. Bend over and reach arms out in front of you, locking thumbs, as if preparing to dive. Breathe. Repeat five times. Relax in this posture, let go of worries and cravings. Reach down and touch the ground with gratitude, as an act of surrender. Let go of your need to consume more and more.

Lap Cradle: Collapse into your lap, cradling your head in your knees. Put hands out, as if diving, then let them drop to your sides or hug your thighs. Breathe and relax. With each exhale, surrender more to gravity. If your head does not reach your thighs comfortably, put a pillow or folded jacket in your lap.

Meditation for cravings: Look beyond the actual object of your craving to see what you actually crave. All addictions are about sensation. Unless you can learn to observe sensation, you can't control craving.

An excellent awakening to sensations is available through practicing Vipassana meditation (see glossary). Indian sage Sri Aurobindo wrote, ―The rejection of the object ceases to be necessary when the object can no longer ensnare us because what the soul enjoys is no longer the object as an object but the Divine which it expresses.‖

When you crave something to consume, food, sex, drink, recognize you are trying to numb yourself from pain. Overdoing is one way we attempt to suffocate fear and all its cousins: anger, ignorance, pain, doubt, lust and the like. When we have a powerful craving for sweets, this addiction often points out that we want something sweet in our life that is missing.

We don't need to go to the opposite extreme of addiction and renounce everything. Rather, we need to find our balance, between the two extremes, what Buddha called, ―the middle way,‖ what our mothers called, ―moderation.‖ Addiction often occurs because we will do anything to not feel. Fear of our own company is rooted in a larger fear that we are not good enough.

Those who are obsessed with relationships, addicted to relationships, use loving someone else as a great distraction from their own company. Male sex addicts follow their penis around like a pointer, like it is their chauffeur. Where are you taking me today? Stuck in the needs and identity of the second *chakra*, sex addicts are all about satisfying basic sensory needs. Called playboys, these men continue to play as boys, never growing up.

Once you become aware that life has a more beautiful dimension beyond the sensory level, you get freedom from the pairs of opposites, the cravings and the aversions. As an addict, once you decide it is time to make a change, a wise place to start is giving up anything unlawful.

Diet: Regardless of what substance or behavior one is addicted to, alter the diet to stop cravings and urges. Eat a fresh, light diet with lots of green vegetables, and few spices or fats.

ANEMIA

Bellows Breath: Two minutes of amplified, normal nose breathing. If you want to draw energy from above, imagine your breath is following a garland from your crown *chakra* down the front of the body through every *chakra*. At the root *chakra*, you begin to exhale up the garland on the back of the body, ending at the crown and begin again. If you wish to draw energy from the earth, begin the inhale at the root *chakra*, coming up to crown, with exhale going down back to root *chakra* and begin again. This breath can be gradually speeded up, and the length of time increased from two minutes, to fan the heat or fire.

Shining Skull: Close eyes and mouth, breathe only through nose. Take a few deep breaths to prepare. As you exhale, imagine you are snuffing a fly off your nose. The forced exhale feels like a short burst of breath, causing your abdominal muscles to contract briefly and your diaphragm to move down.

Optionally, place your hands on belly, and feel your stomach pumping or jumping quickly. No inhale action required; this is called passive breathing. Repeat snuffing and pumping, one exhale per second. Start with three rounds of 20 to 30 pumpings. Gradually increase to 60 pumpings, one minute.

Alternate Nostril Breathing: Hold right hand up to nose, with elbow slightly tucked to your side and shoulder relaxed. Left hand resting on thigh. Gently close right nostril with right thumb and inhale from the left. Close left nostril with ring finger and exhale from right. Keep left nostril closed and inhale from right. Close right nostril with thumb and exhale from left. These steps comprise one round. Retention of breath can be added between each inhale and exhale, to promote the development of muscle mass.

Rolled Pipe Tongue Cooling Breath: Roll tongue like a pipe, stick out of mouth and inhale, drawing air over tongue. If you can't roll your tongue, this is actually an inherited talent, do the *Hissing Breath*: Slightly open mouth, with teeth slightly parted and tongue planted behind lower teeth and inhale. For both styles of cooling breath, after inhaling, swallow and exhale through left nostril, holding right nostril closed with right thumb. Repeat five-eight times.

Furnace Breath: Inhale making soft snoring noise in throat, like a baby sleeping. Swallow to hold breath. Exhale from left nostril only, holding right closed with right thumb. Do eight complete cycles. Removes phlegm from the throat and improves digestion.

Seated Forward Bend: In chair, extend legs out in front of you and reach out to touch toes, dropping forehead toward knees. Hang and breathe. Repeat 3-5 times.

Elbow Pumping: Sit, pump arms up and down, hands in fists. Activates heart and other organs, helps make blood.

Diet: Fresh fruit and dark green, leafy vegetables.

ANGER

When anger is stored, it not only festers but creates disease. Many angry people say they cannot cry, that they haven't cried since they were children. Angry people, find a way to cry! Rent a sad movie or read a sad book and allow the tears to flow.

Fire Essence Breath: Exhale and tuck chin against neck/chest in chin lock. Rapidly pump the belly inside (contract and expand abdominal muscles). Try three rounds of 10 pumpings per round, to start. Inhale and exhale after each round. Build up to 60-100 pumpings per round. Cleans up digestive disorders, constipation, strengthens abdomen. Best with empty stomach and bowels. *Do not do if more than three months pregnant.* Excellent after delivery, to tighten up pelvic and abdominal muscles. Proven to help flatten the abdomen.

Humming Bee Breath: Three fingers placed not pressed on eyeballs, thumbs in ears. Inhale. On the exhale say Om, with five percent of the exhaled sound O of the Om and 95 percent of the exhaled sound the M. Concentrate on third eye and crown *chakra*. Sounds like a powerful bee has taken over the inside of the head. India's black bees are gigantic, patent leather doll shoes hovering over the mango flowers. As a Westerner, I think the Humming Bee sounds more like an 18-wheeler truck blasting its horn to warn of a head on collision.

Rolled Pipe Tongue Cooling Breath: Roll tongue like a pipe, stick out of mouth and inhale, drawing air over tongue. If you can't roll your tongue, this is actually an inherited talent, do the *Hissing Breath*: Slightly open mouth, with teeth slightly parted and tongue planted behind lower teeth and inhale. For both styles of cooling breath, after inhaling, swallow and exhale through left nostril, holding right nostril closed with right thumb. Repeat five-eight times.

Shining Skull: Close eyes and mouth, breathe only through nose. Take a few deep breaths to prepare. As you exhale, imagine you are snuffing a fly off your nose. The forced exhale feels like a short burst of breath, causing your abdominal muscles to contract briefly and your diaphragm to move down. Optionally, place your hands on belly, and feel your stomach pumping or jumping quickly. No inhale action required; this is called passive breathing. Repeat snuffing and pumping, one exhale per second. Start with three rounds of 20 to 30 pumpings. Gradually increase to 60 pumpings, one minute.

Furnace or Victorious Breath: Inhale making soft snoring noise in throat, like a baby sleeping. Swallow to hold breath. Exhale from left nostril only, holding right closed with right thumb. Do eight complete cycles. Removes phlegm from the throat and improves digestion.

Anger is stored in various parts of the body, but most

commonly in the lungs, stomach and calves. Most yoga poses for anger involve stretching or squeezing the stomach and calves.

Seated camel: Sit upright in a low backed chair or on a stool. Reach behind you and sit on your hands, fingers pointed forward, palm down. Arch back, drop head back and open chest, leaning over back of chair. Inhale and exhale deeply and slowly.

Psychic Union: Sit with eyes closed. Hold wrist with other hand behind back. Inhale deeply. When exhaling, fall forward, spine straight, bringing forehead as close to lap as possible. Stay and breathe as long as comfortable. Do once more, changing which hand is gripping and being gripped.

Seated Forward Bend: Sit with legs straight out in front, knees not bent, toes pointed upwards. Reaching out of the hips and shoulders, inhale deeply as you reach up high. On the slow exhale reach out in front of you (not collapsing) toward toes. Grab toes, ankles, shins or any part of legs you can comfortably reach. Breathe comfortably, letting the leg muscles stretch. Relax your back. Drop forehead to knees. Hold breath for five seconds. Return to starting position, do as many as comfortable.

Get Off My Back: Place clenched fists beside bottom of ribcage. Lift elbows up as high as you can behind you, then swing fists forward. Swing forward and back, adding the audio, ―Get off my back‖ in loud staccato bursts with your breath, each time you pull the elbows back. Feel the release.

Legal Tantrum: Sit and stomp feet, like an irate member of the marching band. Enjoy it. Become an irate drum major, and kick one leg forward at a time, with gusto. Like a two year old, you can dump lots of anger with this simple action. Do as long as it feels good.

Meditation: If you are angry with another person, get a photo of them before age 5, and focus on this picture, meditating on the pure child they still are. Imagine you could be wrong, that you made a correct observation of the situation, but drew the wrong conclusion or interpretation. When you consider this possibility, you learn the distinction between knowledge and understanding.

I once freaked out while walking on a dusty Indian road, thinking something dangerous had a hold of my ankles. A thorny branch had gotten caught in the hem of my long skirt, and when I walked it felt like I had been grabbed. By changing my conclusion, I released my fear and anger.

Be careful you don't become the person you dislike, in your efforts to make a case against them. See that the one who makes you angry is most like a disowned part of yourself. Get in touch with that shadow you deny or ignore in you.

One of my most angry moments as an adult came on quite suddenly, toward an obese woman I was rooming with, who did little more than eat in bed and then sleep. We had volunteered to help a nonprofit organization, and had a tremendous amount of work to do, but she was doing virtually nothing. Until I acknowledged there was a part of me that just wanted to stay in bed, eat and sleep, gain weight and avoid responsibility, I remained furious with my roommate.

By accepting the hidden sides of ourselves, we can defuse and neutralize the anger we feel toward the other person. Thank them; they are just your proxy!

Once you become aware or awake to this truth, you see that events and people merely give you opportunity to dump some anger you are holding or generating.

When a tree doesn't grow well, the gardener doesn't get angry at it. The tree isn't blamed for dying. Yet, we blame others, our children and our spouses, when things aren't going the way we want. Blame and anger aren't the answer. Stored anger is linked to a variety of diseases, cancer being one of them. Think of how the language of cancer and anger is shared: both fester, both are stored, both eat at us.

Do you want to be right or healthy? When I was 15 sitting in a driver's education class, my teacher, Reese Protz, presented a scenario for our discussion. —If you are driving down the road, clearly with the right of way, and a car that does not have the right of way enters your lane from the side, do you slow down or keep your speed?‖

A student answered, —If you have the right of way, you can keep going!‖

Mr. Protz answered, —Then that's what they'll put on your

tombstone, _He had the right of way.'‖

Do you want to be right or alive and happy? Do you want to remain angry or embody peace?

The problem is, we all want peace, as long as we can have the last word or can throw the last bomb! The way to assure peace is for us to stop the fighting. As a Buddhist monk, Thich Nhat Hanh teaches it is all about reconciliation, not victory.

Throughout the corrections systems in the US, a model called restorative justice is springing up, to settle disputes. Based on an aboriginal method for restoring community following a crime, the process reminds the doer of a bad deed of all of his goodness, showing him the consequences of his actions, and allows him a chance to make right, to redeem himself and the situation.

This practice is very similar to the seven steps of Buddhist reconciliation, as lived for the past 2500 years by monks in monasteries. Buddhists say that everyone we meet has been our mother or father in a previous life. This belief is taught to help us treat others with respect, as it assumes we will treat our parents with respect. If this image doesn't work for you, perhaps can think of everyone having been your child. (See <u>Being Peace</u>, by Thich Nhat Hanh.)

Practicing forgiveness is a wonderful gift to give yourself. After all, you are absolutely the one most aware of your anger, so why not let it go?

When you are holding anger that originated in your childhood, sit your child self in your lap and love him or her; rock him or her, tell her or him what s/he wants and needs to hear. Hold your child until the tears are no more.

ANXIETY, MOODINESS, DEPRESSION AND OTHER NERVOUS DISORDERS

We are full of pairs of opposites. We may present ourselves as a real neatnik who keeps a spotless home, while deep down there is a poor slob, begging to be set free! We need not let the disowned parts of ourselves pull us down.

When you feel low or in a funk, take a moment and search for the value of this moment, when you feel less than cheerful and hopeful. Examine what benefits are coming from your withdrawal from daily life. Perhaps these times of feeling out of control help you apply the brakes when you are spinning out of control?

Wake up to the reality that other people and things are not out to get you, or operating in relation to you. Develop a kind of immunity to people and circumstances; by realizing that you are not the center of the universe, that self-centeredness has put you in the situation you are in now.

Alternate Nostril Breathing: Hold right hand up to nose, with elbow slightly tucked to your side and shoulder relaxed. Left hand resting on thigh. Gently close right nostril with right thumb and inhale from the left. Close left nostril with ring finger and exhale from right. Keep left nostril closed and inhale from right. Close right nostril with thumb and exhale from left. These steps comprise one round. Retention of breath can be added between each inhale and exhale, to promote the development of muscle mass. When practicing to relieve anxiety, concentrate on breathing soft and slow.

Shining Skull (Kapalabhati): Close eyes and mouth, breathe only through nose. Take a few deep breaths to prepare. As you exhale, imagine you are snuffing a fly off your nose. The forced exhale feels like a short burst of breath, causing your abdominal muscles to contract briefly and your diaphragm to move down. Optionally, place your hands on belly, and feel your stomach pumping or jumping quickly. No inhale action required; this is called passive breathing. Repeat snuffing and pumping, one exhale per second. Start with three rounds of 20 to 30 pumpings. Gradually increase to 60 pumpings, one minute.

Bellows Breath: Two minutes of amplified, normal nose breathing. If you want to draw energy from above, imagine your breath is following a garland from your crown *chakra* down the front of the body through every *chakra*. At the root *chakra*, you begin to exhale up the garland on the back of the body, ending at the crown and begin again. If you wish to draw energy from the earth, begin the inhale at the root *chakra*, coming up to crown, with exhale going down back to root *chakra* and begin again. This breath can be gradually speeded up, and the length of time increased from two minutes, to fan the heat or fire.

Humming Bee Breath: Three fingers placed not pressed on eyeballs, thumbs in ears. Inhale. On the exhale say Om, with five percent of the exhaled sound O of the Om and 95 percent of the exhaled sound the M. Concentrate on third eye and crown *chakra*. Sounds like a powerful bee has taken over the inside of the head. India's black bees are gigantic, patent leather doll shoes hovering over the mango flowers. As a Westerner, I think the Humming Bee sounds more like an 18-wheeler truck blasting its horn to warn of a head on collision.

Rolled Pipe Tongue Cooling Breath: Roll tongue like a pipe, stick out of mouth and inhale, drawing air over tongue. If you can't roll your tongue, this is actually an inherited talent, do the *Hissing Breath*: Slightly open mouth, with teeth slightly parted and tongue planted behind lower teeth and inhale. For both styles of cooling breath, after inhaling, swallow and exhale through left nostril, holding right nostril closed with right thumb.

Each breathing exercise can be done for five minutes for tremendous value. *See Chapters 4 and 5 for more information on the breath being our natural tranquilizer.*

Recognizing the strong relationship between the mind and anxious feelings, Yoga encourages the mind to be still, through practicing poses where the head is placed low or on the ground. The comforting heat of one's thighs against the chest also reduces tension.

Psychic Union: Sit with eyes closed. Hold wrist with other hand behind back. Inhale deeply. When exhaling, fall forward, spine straight, bringing forehead as close to lap as possible, arms up behind you. Stay and breathe as long as comfortable. Do once more, changing which hand is gripping and being gripped.

Seated Forward Bend: Sit with legs straight out in front, knees not bent, feet flexed with toes pointed up. Reaching out of the hips and shoulders, inhale deeply as you reach up high. On the slow exhale reach out in front of you (not collapsing) toward toes. Grab toes, ankles, shins or any part of legs you can comfortably reach. Breathe comfortably, letting the leg muscles stretch. Relax your back. Drop forehead to knees. Hold breath for five seconds. Return to starting position, do as many rounds as comfortable.

Lap Cradle: Collapse into your lap, cradling your head in your knees. Put hands out, as if diving, then let them drop to your sides or hug your thighs. Breathe and relax. With each exhale, surrender more to gravity. If your head does not reach your thighs comfortably, put a pillow or folded jacket in your lap.

Seated Tree: Lace fingers in front of body and turn palms outward. Stretch the arms overhead, pulling in a giant breath. Exhale. Repeat up to five times.

Rake and Shake: Place right hand near or above left shoulder blade. Support right elbow with left hand. Using right hand, look for pain in your should blade area. Squeeze, poke, pinch, knead, rub. Use four strong fingers and rake from shoulder blade up over shoulder, then shake off the pain from your hand and repeat. Reverse sides and use left hand on right shoulder blade.

Get off my back: Place clenched fists beside the bottom of your ribcage. Lift elbows up as high as you can behind you, then swing fists forward. Swing forward and back, adding the audio, —Get off my back‖ in loud staccato bursts with your breath, each time you pull the elbows back. Feel the release.

Meditation: Depression can sometimes be what we feel when we are too polite to admit we are angry or bitter. Women especially find expressing anger difficult, and unconsciously opt for the socially more appropriate mood of depression. Perhaps you need to sit and be honest with yourself. Remember, stress is homemade. Are you angry? Do you feel someone owes you an apology? Do you need to forgive yourself? *Read the section on anger, particularly the meditation, and see if it feels right.*

Examine what throws you out of bed in the morning. Is it love or fear? What motivates you, excitement about creating something or fear of failure? If it is fear, stay in bed until you can hear love calling you.

See yourself as a leaf, floating on the river. Find a place you feel safe and sit or lie down comfortably. Go with the flow of the river; enjoy the safe experience of doing nothing and being okay.

Remaining in this state of ease, tense and relax your feet,

thighs, buttocks, stomach, hands, shoulder, neck and throat, face. Start at face and reverse the process, tensing and relaxing from top to bottom. See the power you have over how much tension you choose to hold or release.

Diet: Certain foods are known to increase mood elevating brain chemicals. A small amount of walnuts, almonds and sunflower seeds can bring a great lift, when the blues hit. Calcium is also concerned a mineral for lifting the spirits, so how about a hot cup of milk with honey?

ARMS, HANDS, WEAK WRISTS CARPAL TUNNEL

Halt: Put right arm straight out in front of you, with hand up, as if you are saying, —halt!‖ With other hand, pull fingertips back and release. Do three times. Then let right hand turn, so fingers are pointing downward and again, using left hand, pull fingers back, 3 times. Repeat with other arm.

Hand Curl: Put both arms out in front and curl hands down and then flip hands back up so fingers are pointing upwards.

Wrist Rolls: Sit with hands in fists, thumbs next to each other. Begin rolling fists in circles, keeping hands in contact with each other, as hands rise up in front of you and go over head, then reverse direction of roll and come back down. Do again and this time when overhead, split hands apart and have them roll down solo, with arms extended out to sides and back to lap.

Pushing Prayer: Put hands in prayer position, in front of chest, elbows straight out to side. Using resistance, press hand and fingers against the other, keeping arms still. Do for 2 minutes.

Finger Push-ups: Put hands in prayer position, separate palms while pointing the fingers at each other and touching all fingertips to each other. Bring hands together; extending fingers flat so they touch each other, then pull back so only tips touch. Repeat 20 times. Flip left hand so palm is facing up; repeat with right hand on top, sometimes known as —spider on the mirror‖! Do 20 times, flip left hand so it is on top with palm facing down and repeat.

Fist and Flower: Inhale, clench fists tightly with thumb inside and hold breath, in the symbol of hostility. Exhale, open palms and fingers wide, in the symbol of hospitality. Repeat.

Back and Forth: Sit straight, reach back with both arms and grab back of chair. Keep holding chair and lean back, stretch pectorals and upper arms, then lean forward over knees, continuing to hold back of chair. Pulse back and forth in small movement.

Squeeze and Tremble: Clasp hands together with arms partially extended directly in front of the chest, elbows slightly bent. Inhale as you squeeze hands together, pressing palms together as well as the space between fingers. It is normal to feel a tremble. Repeat five to eight times, wait 5 or 10 minutes and repeat indefinitely.

ARTHRITIS

Humming Bee Breath: Three fingers placed not pressed on eyeballs, thumbs in ears. Inhale. On the exhale say Om, with five percent of the exhaled sound O of the Om and 95 percent of the exhaled sound the M. Concentrate on third eye and crown *chakra*. Sounds like a powerful bee has taken over the inside of the head. India's black bees are gigantic, patent leather doll shoes hovering over the mango flowers. As a Westerner, I think the Humming Bee sounds more like an 18-wheeler truck blasting its horn to warn of a head on collision.

Shining Skull (Kapalabhati): Close eyes and mouth, breathe only through nose. Take a few deep breaths to prepare. As you exhale, imagine you are snuffing a fly off your nose. The forced exhale feels like a short burst of breath, causing your abdominal muscles to contract briefly and your diaphragm to move down. Optionally, place your hands on belly, and feel your stomach pumping or jumping quickly. No inhale action required; this is called passive breathing. Repeat snuffing and pumping, one exhale per second. Start with three rounds of 20 to 30 pumpings. Gradually increase to 60 pumpings, one minute.

Begin with *Toe to Top Light Warm Ups*, at opening of this chapter. Good for bursitis, too.

Squeeze and Tremble: Clasp hands together with arms partially extended directly in front of the chest, elbows slightly bent. Inhale as you squeeze hands together, pressing palms together as well as the space between fingers. It is normal to feel a tremble. Repeat five to eight times, wait 5 or 10 minutes and repeat indefinitely.

Meditation: Consider how your thinking as well as your body has become inflexible. Reflect on ways you can become less rigid and more flexible in your thinking and actions. Become aware of moments when you are hard on yourself and others and lighten up. Close your eyes and see yourself as a dancing firefly, moving through the air, effortlessly, easily negotiating your way, being a delight to all who see you.

Diet: Deal with constipation. Stop eating meat, excess protein deposits are being stored in your joints. *See Chapter 8 on Constipation.*

Dr. Nedungadi says that those who walk like a cow (with a stiff gate, bent over) have eaten too much cow.

BACKACHE

Furnace Breath: Inhale making soft snoring noise in throat, like a baby sleeping. Swallow to hold breath. Exhale from left nostril only, holding right closed with right thumb. Do eight complete cycles. Removes phlegm from the throat and improves digestion.

Humming Bee Breath: Three fingers placed not pressed on eyeballs, thumbs in ears. Inhale. On the exhale say Om, with five percent of the exhaled sound *O* of the Om and 95 percent of the exhaled sound the *M*. Concentrate on third eye and crown *chakra*. Sounds like a powerful bee has taken over the inside of the head. India's black bees are gigantic, patent leather doll shoes hovering over the mango flowers. As a Westerner, I think the Humming Bee sounds more like an 18-wheeler truck blasting its horn to warn of a head on collision.

Get off my back, for upper back: Place clenched fists beside bottom of ribcage. Lift elbows up as high as you can behind you, then swing fists forward. Swing forward and back, adding the audio, —Get off my back‖ in loud staccato bursts with your breath, each time you pull the elbows back. Feel the release. (For more upper back help, see Shoulder section.)

Knee Squeeze: Pull one knee at a time up to chest. Squeeze. Repeat four or more times with each leg. Then pull and hold both knees at chest.

Hold and Release Beach Ball: Imagine you are holding a giant beach ball, so large it makes your chest cave in to hold it. Exhale fully to better get a hold of the ball. Suddenly, take a great inhale and pull your outstretched arms back as far as you can, puffing up the chest and letting the ball go. Repeat up to five times.

Grinding Wheel: Clasp hands together, imagining they are holding the handle of a large wheel that is parallel to the floor. Sit on the edge of your chair. Reach far out to your left and pull the wheel all the way to the right, then lean back and bring your clasped hands to your chest, then swing out wide to the left again. Grind five complete circles in one direction, then reverse. Inhale as you reach out and exhale as you bring the hands toward the chest.

Seated Rowboat: Sit on edge of seat. If comfortable doing so, hold legs off the ground, straight out in front of you. (If not, keep feet on floor) Hold your imaginary oars, palms down and exhale as you extend the arms fully, reaching forward, as far as comfortable. Lean back, exhale and pull elbows back as far as you can. The hands are making a circle as you row. Repeat five to 10 times.

Seated Cat Stretch: Standing or sitting, place hands on thighs. Inhale, raise head and drop it back. Push the chest forward, arching back. Hold a few seconds. Exhale while dropping chin to chest, pulling stomach in and squeezing all air out of body, humping the back like a scared cat. Hold a few seconds. Do five to 10 rounds, with slow breath.

Seated Tree and Swaying Tree: Lace fingers in front of body and turn palms outward. Stretch the arms overhead, pulling in a giant breath. Exhale and bend at the waist to the right. Inhale as you come back up to center, exhale to the left. Repeat up to five times, each side.

Seated Twist: Sit upright. Reach right arm across chest and reach behind left shoulder to hold back of chair, sliding hand along back of chair as far to right as possible. Keep fanny on seat. Turn head and look over right shoulder and continue to breathe. Take two complete breaths. Reverse, using left arm. Repeat up to five times on each side.

Seated Camel: Sit upright in a low backed chair or on a stool. Reach behind you and sit on your hands, fingers pointed forward, palm down. Arch back, drop head back and open chest, leaning over back of chair. Inhale and exhale deeply and slowly.

Diet: Avoid overeating and heavy foods. Your back isn't made to carry more than your frame is designed to carry. Are you carrying the weight of the world? Drop some weight and feel better.

Meditation: Look at what is bothering you back there, what you need to let go of that is now behind you. The past is the past; it is time to be free of that pain. Perhaps your pain is due to believing something was done behind your back, a betrayal, being stabbed in the back. Let this thought go, it is hurting you. Is there a shield behind your heart that you can release?

Look at where you might need more support in your life and create it for yourself. Are you being upstanding in your own life, upholding yourself, giving yourself needed support, good posture and positive thinking?

BLOOD PRESSURE, HIGH

Hypertension affects one in ten Indians, and has been steadily increasing as a major health problem in India for the past 50 years. If left untreated, hypertension raises the risk of heart attack, congestive heart failure and stroke. Chronic diseases are a leading cause of death in India. —At least 80 percent of premature heart disease, stroke and type two diabetes, and 40 percent of cancer (could be) prevented through a healthy diet, regular physical exercise and avoiding tobacco products, according to the World Health Organization.

Hypertension affects over 50 million Americans, or nearly one in four adults. If left untreated, hypertension raises the risk of heart attack, congestive heart failure and stroke. Cardiovascular diseases are responsible for more deaths each year than the next seven leading causes of death combined. According to the American Heart Association, only 27 percent of people with high blood pressure have their disease under control.

Yogis have long known that lifestyle influences health. Even talking raises blood pressure, and exhaling lowers it. According to a study conducted at Rush Presbyterian St. Luke's Medical Center, —Slow and deep breathing is well known to regulate both cardiovascular and nervous systems. The greater lung inflation associated with deep and slow breathing stimulates slowly adapting pulmonary stretch receptors in the cells of the lungs, which leads to blood pressure reduction.‖ (www.rush.edu)

For every excessive pound of weight we carry, the body adds another mile of blood vessels and a point to the upper number of the blood pressure. With more mass to feed with blood, the body must send blood out further from the heart, requiring it to push through miles more of vessels.

Alternate Nostril Breathing: Hold right hand up to nose, with elbow slightly tucked to your side and shoulder relaxed. Left hand resting on thigh. Gently close right nostril with right thumb and inhale from the left. Close left nostril with ring finger and exhale from right. Keep left nostril closed and inhale from right. Close right nostril with thumb and exhale from left. These steps comprise one round. Retention of breath can be added between each inhale and exhale, to promote the development of muscle mass. Do very slowly with no sound, to relax and lower pressure.

Rolled Pipe Tongue Cooling Breath: Roll tongue like a pipe, stick out of mouth and inhale, drawing air over tongue. If you can't roll your tongue (an inherited talent), do the *Hissing Breath*: Slightly open mouth, with teeth slightly parted and tongue planted behind lower teeth and inhale. For both styles of cooling breath, after inhaling, swallow and exhale through left nostril, holding right nostril closed with right thumb. Repeat five-eight times.

Furnace Breath: Inhale making soft snoring noise in throat, like a baby sleeping. Swallow to hold breath. Exhale from left nostril only, holding right closed with right thumb. Do eight complete cycles. Removes phlegm from the throat and improves digestion.

Humming Bee Breath: Three fingers placed not pressed on eyeballs, thumbs in ears. Inhale. On the exhale say Om, with five percent of the exhaled sound O of the Om and 95 percent of the exhaled sound the M. Concentrate on third eye and crown *chakra*. Sounds like a powerful bee has taken over the inside of the head. India's black bees are gigantic, patent leather doll shoes hovering over the mango flowers. As a Westerner, I think the Humming Bee sounds more like an 18-wheeler truck blasting its horn to warn of a head on collision. Alternate Nostril Breathing, Furnace Breath and Humming Bee Breath are also good for regulating low pressure).

Most of our circulatory system runs close to the bones, so we cannot touch or feel the flow of blood. One spot on the body we can feel the movement of blood is at the wrist, where we feel both an artery and veins. By simply squeezing the wrists and fingertips, we affect blood flow.

Light Warm Ups, see opening of this chapter.

Squeeze and Chant: At pulse point, hold your wrist tight with opposite hand wrapping underneath and up around wrist. The fingers are touching the artery and the thumb is touching a vein. You are stopping the flow of blood. Yogis silently chant to the God Rama, ―Sri Ram, Jai Ram, Jai Jai Ram‖ five times to time the squeeze, then pause. The chant means ―Hail God.‖ You can chant it or find another four second phrase (Happy birthday to you, happy birthday to you). Do both wrists. No one can hold your wrist or chant for you, this must be done for yourself by yourself.

Clump and Press: Hold hands in front of you with fingers facing each other. Clump all fingers together and press the tips against each other. The fingertips are the turning point of the circulatory system, so applying pressure slows the blood flow and allows it to reset itself. Practice for one-two minutes. You can also sit and press fingertips down into the chair seat.

Press and Roll: With palm facing up, use other hand to press the ends of each finger with thumb, rolling down from top of finger to first crease on finger. Flip hand over and do same procedure. Repeat on other hand. Like pressing a tube of toothpaste, done to regulate pressure.

Diet: Chew two cardamom pods and swallow the juice. Keep remaining seed in mouth and makes more saliva to swallow. It is cooling, regulates the pressure. Eating raw celery also reduces blood pressure. Reduce overall caloric intake if overweight. Eat vegetarian.

Meditation: Be aware of your circulation. If symptoms arise, such as profuse and sudden sweatiness, heaviness or heavy breathing, hold your own wrist and check your pulse. Feeling the pulse or life force is like touching the Divine, we can't see it, we can only feel it. Thinking is a major cause of high blood pressure, so by controlling the mind and calming stress, blood pressure can be regulated. (Read meditation in Anxiety section.)

BLOOD PRESSURE, LOW AND WEAK HEART

Alternate Nostril Breathing: Hold right hand up to nose, with elbow slightly tucked to your side and shoulder relaxed. Left hand resting on thigh. Gently close right nostril with right thumb and inhale from the left. Close left nostril with ring finger and exhale from right. Keep left nostril closed and inhale from right. Close right nostril with thumb and exhale from left. These steps comprise one round. Retention of breath can be added between each inhale and exhale, to promote the development of muscle mass.

Fire Essence Breath: Exhale and tuck chin against neck/chest in chin lock. Rapidly pump the belly inside (contract and expand abdominal muscles). Try three rounds of 10 pumpings per round, to start. Inhale and exhale after each round. Build up to 60-100 pumpings per round. Cleans up digestive orders, constipation, strengthens abdomen. Best with empty stomach and bowels. *Do not do if more than three months pregnant.* Excellent after delivery, to tighten up pelvic and abdominal muscles. Proven to help flatten the abdomen.

Furnace Breath: Inhale making soft snoring noise in throat, like a baby sleeping. Swallow to hold breath. Exhale from left nostril only, holding right closed with right thumb. Do eight complete cycles. Removes phlegm from the throat and improves digestion.

Bellows Breath: Two minutes of amplified, normal nose breathing. If you want to draw energy from above, imagine your breath is following a garland from your crown *chakra* down the front of the body through every *chakra*. At the root *chakra*, you begin to exhale up the garland on the back of the body, ending at the crown and begin again. If you wish to draw energy from the earth, begin the inhale at the root *chakra*, coming up to crown, with exhale going down back to root *chakra* and begin again. This breath can be gradually speeded up, and the length of time increased from two minutes, to fan the heat or fire.

Shining Skull (Kapalabhati): Close eyes and mouth, breathe only through nose. Take a few deep breaths to prepare. As you exhale, imagine you are snuffing a fly off your nose. The forced exhale feels like a short burst of breath, causing your abdominal muscles to contract briefly and your diaphragm to move down. Optionally, place your hands on belly, and feel your stomach pumping or jumping quickly. No inhale action required; this is called passive breathing. Repeat snuffing and pumping, one exhale per second. Start with three rounds of 20 to 30 pumpings. Gradually increase to 60 pumpings, one minute.

Humming Bee Breath: Three fingers placed not pressed on eyeballs, thumbs in ears. Inhale. On the exhale say Om, with five percent of the exhaled sound O of the Om and 95 percent of the exhaled sound the M. Concentrate on third eye and crown *chakra*. Sounds like a powerful bee has taken over the inside of the head. India's black bees are gigantic, patent leather doll shoes hovering over the mango flowers. As a Westerner, I think the Humming Bee sounds more like an 18-wheeler truck blasting its horn to warn of a head on collision.

Heating Sun Breath: With right hand, use thumb to close right nostril and ring finger to close left. Inhale through right and exhale through left, repeatedly. Especially good in cold weather when you need to feel warmer.

Alternate Nostril Breathing, Furnace Breath and Humming Bee Breath regulate both high and low pressure.

Elbow Pumping: Sit, pump arms up and down, hands in fists. Activates heart and other organs, helps make blood. Practice any poses in this book, dynamically.

Clump and Press: Hold hands in front of you with fingers facing each other. Clump all fingers together and press the tips against each other. The fingertips are the turning point of the circulatory system, so applying pressure slows the blood flow and allows it to reset itself. Practice for one-two minutes. You can also sit and press fingertips down into the chair seat.

Diet: Keep clove in mouth, chew and create saliva to swallow. Eat vegetarian.

CHRONIC PAIN

Any and all breathing exercises work! Find the one that provides the greatest getaway. Counting breaths can help distract the mind and body.

Find the breathing exercise that provides the most mental and physical relief. Squeezing out tension can be especially valuable.

Meditation: Make sure you include the site of your chronic pain while doing this meditation. If it isn't mentioned, simply add to the section that geographically covers your pain.

Sit comfortably with spine straight. Imagine a clear sparkling stream or waterfall of cool water pouring into the top of your head. Let the water fill your head, washing away all excess thoughts and worries. Notice what you are thinking about and enjoy throwing away old thoughts or beliefs that no serve you. Save the thoughts worth keeping for another time. Leave the head; see the brain, eyes, ears and nose sparkling and clean, free of all imperfections. Inhale and exhale. Forgive. Feel this part of your body healed, energized yet relaxed. Be grateful.

Feel the water move down through your throat, neck and shoulders. Feel the water get warmer, and relax the tension in your muscles and joints. Words or feelings you wished you said or hadn't said may come to mind. Let your whole throat be washed, and all wishes washed away. Visualize the neck shoulders, throat, tonsils, jaw, tongue, saliva and thyroid shining brightly with health and well-being. Inhale and exhale. Forgive. Feel this part of your body healed, energized yet relaxed. Be grateful.

Watch the water fill your chest, opening your heart and lungs to cleansing and release. Breathe deeply, exhaling sadness and that sense of a heavy heart. Allow love to fill you. Flood your arms and legs with this cleansing water. Leaving the chest, see the blood, lymph, thymus, heart, lungs, ribs and spine wiped clean of waste, toxins and infection. Inhale and exhale. Forgive. Feel this part of your body healed, energized yet relaxed. Be grateful.

As the water continues to flow down into your abdominal cavity, the center of your being or Solar Plexus, let go and wash out old self images that made you feel small or inadequate. Allow your true radiance to be set free. Leaving the abdomen, see the stomach, liver, pancreas, spleen and gallbladder working perfectly, freed of complications and disturbances. Inhale and exhale. Forgive. Feel this part of your body healed, energized yet relaxed. Be grateful.

Moving downward below the navel, let the water swirl around inside your hips and pelvis, dislodging waste and sludge that has been blocking your emotions, especially your healthy expression of sexuality. Leaving the ovaries, testes, uterus and intestines, notice how you are able to empty your body of all the old, dead matter, the drift wood that has been holding you down and back. Inhale and exhale. Forgive. Feel this part of your body healed, energized yet relaxed. Be grateful.

Finally, watch the steady flow of healing water flow all the way to the tail bone, seeing it draining the body of all pain, tension, insecurity, disappointment, worry, fear, anger, greed and jealousy. Empty yourself of all the baggage and extra weight you have carried unknowingly and unnecessarily. Feel your entire nervous system, from crown to tailbone, flow freely and harmoniously. Flood your legs and feet with refreshing relief. Inhale and exhale. Forgive. Feel this part of your body healed, energized yet relaxed. Be grateful.

After a quick scan to confirm the water has swept you clean, inhale golden healing light from the top of your head down to your toes. On the exhale, send the light back up the body to be released from the top of the head. Embrace your healthy body, knowing it houses only energies that are good for you. Declare you are strong and well, recovering from whatever has been ailing you. Give thanks for the healing and easing into good health. Inhale and exhale. Feel your whole body healed, energized yet relaxed.

COLD OR RUNNY NOSE, ALLERGY, ASTHMA, BRONCHITIS, COUGH, HEADACHE WITH COLD

A strong yoga practice assists in draining lymph and opening up the lungs and throat, to speed up recovery from illness, injury or surgery.

Heating Sun Breath: With right hand, use thumb to close right nostril and ring finger to close left. Inhale through right and exhale through left, repeatedly. Especially good in cold weather when you need to feel warmer.

Bellows Breath: Two minutes of amplified, normal nose breathing. If you want to draw energy from above, imagine your breath is following a garland from your crown *chakra* down the front of the body through every *chakra*. At the root *chakra*, you begin to exhale up the garland on the back of the body, ending at the crown and begin again. If you wish to draw energy from the earth, begin the inhale at the root *chakra*, coming up to crown, with exhale going down back to root *chakra* and begin again. This breath can be gradually speeded up, and the length of time increased from two minutes, to fan the heat or fire.

Furnace Breath: Inhale making soft snoring noise in throat, like a baby sleeping. Swallow to hold breath. Exhale from left nostril only, holding right closed with right thumb. Do eight complete cycles. Removes phlegm from the throat and improves digestion.

Alternate Nostril Breathing: Hold right hand up to nose, with elbow slightly tucked to your side and shoulder relaxed. Left hand resting on thigh. Gently close right nostril with right thumb and inhale from the left. Close left nostril with ring finger and exhale from right. Keep left nostril closed and inhale from right. Close right nostril with thumb and exhale from left. These steps comprise one round. Retention of breath can be added between each inhale and exhale, to promote the development of muscle mass. *Humming Bee Breath:* Inhale through nose, shut your eyes and exhale through mouth, making a noise from the back of the throat like a bee (often immediate results). Concentrate on exhaling through the mouth, slowly with sound, heating the breath and killing germs.

For asthma, follow recommended breathing exercises for Anxiety. For colds, do no strenuous yoga poses.

Seated Cat Stretch: Standing or sitting, place hands on thighs. Inhale, raise head and drop it back. Push the chest forward, arching the back. Hold a few seconds. Exhale while dropping chin to chest, pulling stomach in and squeezing all air out of body, humping the back like a scared cat. Hold a few seconds. Do five to 10 rounds, with slow breath.

Seated Rag Doll: Sit. While inhaling, raise arms above head with limp wrists. Swing down to the floor with a forced exhale, even adding a grunt or sound from deep in the belly like —hah! to fully empty lungs. If hands touch floor, bring them back behind feet as far as possible. Hang loose with head in lap! Repeat up to five times.

Fingers Laced Behind Back: Sitting or standing, lace fingers behind back and fall forward, lifting arms up behind you. Look forward, not down. Repeat up to five times.

Crossed Hands Raised: Tying the breath to the movement of the arms, begin with hands crossed hanging in front. Inhale and raise arms overhead, again crossing hands over the head. Drop head back to look up at hands. Exhale and bring arms out to sides, straight out from shoulders. Inhale back above head, crossed hands. Exhale swing arms down and hang crossed hands in front of body. Repeat entire cycle five to 10 times.

Knee Squeeze: Pull one knee at a time up to chest. Squeeze. Repeat four or more times with each leg. Then pull and hold both knees at chest.

Seated Tree: Lace fingers in front of body and turn palms outward. Stretch the arms overhead, pulling in a giant breath. Exhale. Repeat up to five times.

Seated Camel. Sit upright in a low backed chair or on a stool. Reach behind you and sit on your hands, fingers pointed forward, palm down. Arch back, drop head back and open chest, leaning over back of chair. Inhale and exhale deeply and slowly.

Head Rolling: Place top of head on flat surface of desk or table, palms flat on desktop. Roll the head around, releasing the stress and pain. If it feels good to do so, stand up and continue rolling the head on the desktop.

Diet: Avoid dairy products (mucus producing), meat and raw vegetables.

Meditation: Reflect on how you are doing too much, and where you can cut back. Look at how you may be thinking that others are out to get you. Make sure you are making choices for your highest good, not being overly influenced by others or trying to please them.

CONSTIPATION

A system of living, Yoga offers techniques for supporting any and all body functions, and constipation is no exception. *See Chapter 8.*

Fire Essence Breath: Exhale and tuck chin against neck/chest in chin lock. Rapidly pump the belly inside (contract and expand abdominal muscles). Try three rounds of 10 pumpings per round, to start. Inhale and exhale after each round. Build up to 60-100 pumpings per round. Cleans up digestive disorders, constipation, strengthens abdomen. Best on empty stomach and bowel. *Don't do if more than three months pregnant.* Excellent after delivery, to tighten up pelvic and abdominal muscles. Proven to help flatten the abdomen.

Shining Skull: Close eyes and mouth, breathe only through nose. Take a few deep breaths to prepare. As you exhale, imagine you are snuffing a fly off your nose. The forced exhale feels like a short burst of breath, causing your abdominal muscles to contract briefly and your diaphragm to move down. Optionally, place your hands on belly, and feel your stomach pumping or jumping quickly. No inhale action required; this is called passive breathing. Repeat snuffing and pumping, one exhale per second. Start with three rounds of 20 to 30 pumpings. Gradually increase to 60 pumpings, one minute.

Alternate Nostril Breathing: Hold right hand up to nose, with elbow slightly tucked to your side and shoulder relaxed. Left hand resting on thigh. Gently close right nostril with right thumb and inhale from the left. Close left nostril with ring finger and exhale from right. Keep left nostril closed and inhale from right. Close right nostril with thumb and exhale from left. These steps comprise one round. Retention of breath can be added between each inhale and exhale, to promote the development of muscle mass.

If able, pull in and hold stomach in for first two poses.

Knee Squeeze: Pull one knee at a time up to chest. Squeeze. Repeat four or more times with each leg. Then pull and hold both knees at chest. Particularly focus on the left leg, as you squeeze against the descending colon. (Here's a simple cue to remember:

squeeze the left, the Left is where Elvis Leaves the building! Think L, as in Let Go.)

Heel Thumping: (if possible, better done standing) Stand on toes then forcefully bring body weight down on heels. Repeat this strong, focused thump three to five times. The bowel point on the bottom of the foot is being stimulated.

Lap Cradle: Collapse into your lap, cradling your head in your knees. Put hands out, as if diving, then let them drop to your sides or hug your thighs. Breathe and relax. With each exhale, surrender more to gravity. If your head does not reach your thighs comfortably, put a pillow or folded jacket in your lap. If comfortable, suck in and lock belly to encourage intestines.

Seated Camel: Sit upright in a low backed chair or on a stool. Reach behind you and sit on your hands, fingers pointed forward, palm down. Arch back, drop head back and open chest, leaning over back of chair. Inhale and exhale deeply and slowly.

Seated Twist: Sit upright. Take right arm and cross chest and reach behind shoulder to hold back of chair, sliding hand as far to right as possible. Keep fanny on seat. Turn head and look over right shoulder and continue to breathe. Take two complete breaths. Reverse, using left arm. Repeat up to five times.

Seated Rowboat: Sit on edge of seat. If comfortable doing so, hold legs off the ground, straight out in front of you. (If not, keep feet on floor) Hold your imaginary oars, palms down and exhale as you extend the arms fully, reaching forward, as far as comfortable. Lean back, exhale and pull elbows back as far as you can. The hands are making a circle as you row. Repeat five to 10 times.

Wrist squeeze: take one wrist and then the other and vigorously squeeze and twist.

Rectum pulsing (Ashwini): Tighten and squeeze rectum, pulling it up and holding without strain as long as comfortable. Continue, rhythmically tightening and releasing the rectum, and being conscious of not adding other parts of the body such as thighs, buttocks or stomach to pulsation. Do throughout the day, as much as comfortable. Increase speed of contractions as able. Breathe normally.

Meditation: Sitting comfortably, enjoy a deep exhale. As you inhale, feel the lightness of the breath create a sense of weightlessness in your body. As you exhale, allow yourself to release tension, unwanted and unneeded thoughts and other negative energies. Continue to breathe in healing white light. With each exhale, imagine letting go of an activity, piece of personal property or a relationship you are ready to detach from. See the old float away on the smokiness of your exhale. Relax. Release.

DIABETES

Seated camel: Sit upright in a low backed chair or on a stool. Reach behind you and sit on your hands, fingers pointed forward, palm down. Arch back, drop head back and open chest, leaning over back of chair. Inhale and exhale deeply and slowly.

Diet: Diabetes is rising, in India, due to heavy consumption of white rice; in the West due to excessive intake of fats and sugar. Make sure starches are not the largest serving of food on your plate. Vegetables should be the largest food group.

EYESIGHT (FOR TIRED EYES, AS WELL AS TO IMPROVE VISION)

Humming Bee Breath: Three fingers placed not pressed on eyeballs, thumbs in ears. Inhale. On the exhale say Om, with five percent of the exhaled sound O of the Om and 95 percent of the exhaled sound the M. Concentrate on third eye and crown *chakra*. Sounds like a powerful bee has taken over the inside of the head. India's black bees are gigantic, patent leather doll shoes hovering over the mango flowers. As a Westerner, I think the Humming Bee sounds more like an 18-wheeler truck blasting its horn to warn of a head on collision.

Circling Thumbs: With hands clasped together tightly keep thumbs up and circle arms around in front of you, quickly, following your thumbs with eyes. Circle in both directions.

Hitchhiking Thumb: With one arm extended in front of you, follow your thumb slowly, climb up the wall to the ceiling, then move along the ceiling as far as you can bring your arm behind you and still see the thumb. Come back. Reverse hands. Try with thumb moving out to side, again, watch until you can't see it anymore then come back. Repeat several times.

Clock Face: Imagine your face is a clock. Think of random hours, and look at the appropriate area of your face. For example, three o'clock is directly to your right, and 12 is straight up. Move only your eyes. Go in both directions, diagonally and other ways. Breathe slowly and deeply. Strengthens eyes and restores roundness to eyeball. Preferable to do with eyes open.

Thumb Focus: Extend arm in front of you, with thumb up. Focus on the thumbnail, then change your depth of focus and concentrate on the wall or some far location behind the thumb. Go back and forth between the thumbnail and far away point, to sharpen your ability to change focus and depth perception. Repeat with other hand.

Special Practice: Squeeze space between index and middle fingers, kneading and releasing pain. Massage index and middle finger of corresponding eye (left or right).

Meditation: Rub hands together and place warm hands on eyes, fingers pointed up, making a mask over the eyes. Enjoy this energizing hideout for a moment or two. Repeat throughout the day, as needed. With hands lightly on eyes and eyes lightly closed, look for colors. Light colors are a sign of good health. YogaSir encourages you to see pastels, like pink, yellow, white, green and sky blue. Avoid looking for dark colors like black, brown, navy blue.

FALLEN ARCHES

Roll foot on bottle or rolling pin. Try to hold a pen with foot and write, push imaginary marbles with the outside of your foot on the floor and the arch curved like a scoop.

Sitting with feet flat on floor, lift just toes off the floor and hold up. Repeat.

Stand on stairs, drop heels below balls of feet. Alternating come up on toes. Repeat full cycle.

Diet: Drop some weight! Your feet are feeling overwhelmed.

Massage feet nightly with arnica or fragrant essential oil, stretching arch, foot, space between toes.

Fatigue

Shining Skull: Close eyes and mouth, breathe only through nose. Take a few deep breaths to prepare. As you exhale, imagine you are snuffing a fly off your nose. The forced exhale feels like a short burst of breath, causing your abdominal muscles to contract briefly and your diaphragm to move down. Optionally, place your hands on belly, and feel your stomach pumping or jumping quickly. No inhale action required; this is called passive breathing. Repeat snuffing and pumping, one exhale per second. Start with three rounds of 20 to 30 pumpings. Gradually increase to 60 pumpings, one minute.

Alternate Nostril Breathing: Hold right hand up to nose, with elbow slightly tucked to your side and shoulder relaxed. Left hand resting on thigh. Gently close right nostril with right thumb and inhale from the left. Close left nostril with ring finger and exhale from right. Keep left nostril closed and inhale from right. Close right nostril with thumb and exhale from left. These steps comprise one round. Retention of breath can be added between each inhale and exhale, to promote the development of muscle mass.

Humming Bee Breath: Three fingers placed not pressed on eyeballs, thumbs in ears. Inhale. On the exhale say *Om*, with five percent of the exhaled sound *O* of the Om and 95 percent of the exhaled sound the *M*. Concentrate on third eye and crown *chakra*. Sounds like a powerful bee has taken over the inside of the head. India's black bees are gigantic, patent leather doll shoes hovering over the mango flowers. As a Westerner, I think the Humming Bee sounds more like an 18-wheeler truck blasting its horn to warn of a head on collision.

Bellows Breath: Two minutes of amplified, normal nose breathing. If you want to draw energy from above, imagine your breath is following a garland from your crown *chakra* down the front of the body through every *chakra*. At the root *chakra*, you begin to exhale up the garland on the back of the body, ending at the crown and begin again. If you wish to draw energy from the earth, begin the inhale at the root *chakra*, coming up to crown, with exhale going down back to root *chakra* and begin again. This breath can be gradually speeded up, and the length of time increased from two minutes, to fan the heat or fire.

Toe to Top Light Warm Ups, see opening of this chapter.

Knock Knock on Head: With clenched fists, knock knock all over scalp and look for sore spots, which identify tension.

Scalp Shift: Grab hair as close to scalp as possible and pull scalp in all directions. Remember the Wig Hats we wore in the sixties?

Hold and Release Beach Ball: Imagine you are holding a giant beach ball, so large it makes your chest cave in to hold it. Exhale fully to better hold the ball. Suddenly, take a great inhale and pull your outstretched arms back as far as you can, puffing up the chest and letting the ball go. Repeat up to five times.

Meditation: Fatigue can have many causes, particularly poor or improper diet, sleeping habits, worry and anxiety, depression, boredom, repressed anger and workaholic tendencies. When we want to trade our feeling tired for feeling refreshed and energized, it is wise to meditate on the cause of this fatigue. Chasing Shakti (energy) without knowledge is unwise. Reflect on what you might be avoiding. Reflect on what you are looking forward to and feeling enthusiastic about. Ask your body what it needs.

GRIEF

Experiencing grief is a natural part of being human, and it is important to feel loss. Remember that pouring your cup of grief into a larger pot you dilute your pain. This means there is great value in sharing with or telling your grief to others, both those who are also grieving and those who aren't.

Typically held in the chest, grief can be released with:

Chanting Om: To calm down and center. Inhale fully. Say the *O* of the *Om* for 50 percent of the exhale and the *M* for the other 50 percent. Repeat for 5 breaths.

Alternate Nostril Breathing: Hold right hand up to nose, with elbow slightly tucked to your side and shoulder relaxed. Left hand resting on thigh. Gently close right nostril with right thumb and inhale from the left. Close left nostril with ring finger and exhale from right. Keep left nostril closed and inhale from right. Close right nostril with thumb and exhale from left. These steps comprise one round. Retention of breath can be added between each inhale and exhale, to promote the development of muscle mass.

Bellows Breath: Two minutes of amplified, normal nose breathing. If you want to draw energy from above, imagine your breath is following a garland from your crown *chakra* down the front of the body through every *chakra*. At the root *chakra*, you begin to exhale up the garland on the back of the body, ending at the crown and begin again. If you wish to draw energy from the earth, begin the inhale at the root *chakra*, coming up to crown, with exhale going down back to root *chakra* and begin again. This breath can be gradually speeded up, and the length of time increased from two minutes, to fan the heat or fire.

Seated camel: Sit upright in a low backed chair or on a stool. Reach behind you and sit on your hands, fingers pointed forward, palm down. Arch back, drop head back and open chest, leaning over back of chair. Inhale and exhale deeply and slowly.

Hold and Release Beach Ball: Imagine you are holding a giant beach ball, so large it makes your chest cave in to hold it. Exhale fully to better get a hold of the ball. Suddenly, take a great inhale and pull your outstretched arms back as far as you can, puffing up the chest and letting the ball go. Repeat up to five times.

Meditation: As you breathe, see yourself pulling in a lovely healing color, perhaps white or gold like the sun. As you exhale, see your grief leave like smoke on your breath, being carried off into the universe to be purified and recycled. Watch this cycle of breath and see how nature wants to free you of your pain. Recognize the fact that death is a condition of life, and out of our control. Do you really want to be responsible for deciding who and how and when people die? There is rarely a good time for death, in our limited view of the world. We must trust the natural process, the cycle of life.

Second Meditation: Leaning back in your chair, let your head fall behind you and your arms open wide to the sides. Imagine a beautiful, ornate bird cage is your chest. Suddenly, the door pops open and the birds you have had trapped inside for so long are released. Watch them leave…carrying the fear and grief you have held in your chest and heart. Breathe fully and deeply, and exhale in a long slow breath. See the space you have opened up, for new blessings to fly in.

HAIR LOSS

Also address any skin problems on the toes or hands, as there is a relationship to hair loss.

Shining Skull: Close eyes and mouth, breathe only through nose. Take a few deep breaths to prepare. As you exhale, imagine you are snuffing a fly off your nose. The forced exhale feels like a short burst of breath, causing your abdominal muscles to contract briefly and your diaphragm to move down. Optionally, place your hands on belly, and feel your stomach pumping or jumping quickly. No inhale action required; this is called passive breathing. Repeat snuffing and pumping, one exhale per second. Start with three rounds of 20 to 30 pumpings. Gradually increase to 60 pumpings, one minute.

Humming Bee Breath: Three fingers placed not pressed on eyeballs, thumbs in ears. Inhale. On the exhale say *Om*, with five percent of the exhaled sound *O* of the Om and 95 percent of the exhaled sound the *M*. Concentrate on third eye and crown chakra. Sounds like a powerful bee has taken over the inside of the head. India's black bees are gigantic, patent leather doll shoes hovering over the mango flowers. As a Westerner, I think the Humming Bee sounds more like an 18-wheeler truck blasting its horn to warn of a head on collision.

Nail Scrub: Hands face each other, fold over fingers and rub nails of one hand against nails of other hand, creates something like a washboard sound. Go back and forth for a minute or two. Stimulates hair growth.

Neck Release: Drop head between legs and hang. Practice any inversions where the head is lower than the heart, and blood is stimulating the scalp.

Knock Knock on Scalp: with clenched fists, knock knock around scalp and look for sore spots, which identifies tension.

Meditation: Sit comfortably and peacefully, and remind yourself of all the safety and security in your life. Trust the process of life. See meditations in sections for anxiety and skin disorders.

HEADACHE

Bellows Breath: Two minutes of amplified, normal nose breathing. If you want to draw energy from above, imagine your breath is following a garland from your crown *chakra* down the front of the body through every *chakra*. At the root *chakra*, you begin to exhale up the garland on the back of the body, ending at the crown and begin again. If you wish to draw energy from the earth, begin the inhale at the root *chakra*, coming up to crown, with exhale going down back to root *chakra* and begin again. This breath can be gradually speeded up, and the length of time increased from two minutes, to fan the heat or fire.

Rolled Pipe Tongue Cooling Breath: Roll tongue like a pipe, stick out of mouth and inhale, drawing air over tongue. Especially good for migraines. If you can't roll your tongue, this is actually an inherited talent, do the *Hissing Breath*: Slightly open mouth, with teeth slightly parted and tongue planted behind lower teeth and inhale. For both styles of cooling breath, after inhaling, swallow and exhale through left nostril, holding right nostril closed with right thumb. Repeat five-eight times.

If headache is on left side, squeeze arm repeatedly above left elbow for a few moments. If a right side headache, adapt accordingly. If in front of head, rub forehead with fingers pressing up to hairline.

Thumb Rubs: Hold hands, as if twiddling thumbs, gently rub thumbs together.

Squeeze web between thumb and index finger, looking for painful little spot or _bead'. Squeeze and release until pain dissipates in hand.

With hands clasped together tightly keep thumbs up and circle arms around in front of you, quickly, following your thumbs with eyes. Circle in both directions.

Hitchhiking Thumb: With one arm extended in front of you, follow your thumb slowly, climb up the wall to the ceiling, then move along the ceiling as far as you can bring your arm behind you and still see the thumb. Come back. Reverse hands. Try with thumb moving out to side, again, watch until you can't see it anymore then come back. Repeat several times.

Clock Face: Imagine your face is a clock. Think of random hours, and look at the appropriate area of your face. For example, three o'clock is directly to your right, and 12 is straight up. Move only your eyes. Go in both directions, diagonally and other ways. Breathe slowly and deeply. Strengthens eyes and restores roundness to eyeball. Preferable to do with eyes open.

Palming Forehead: with palms facing face, press heels of hands into forehead above brows, sliding all the way up to the hairline. Repeat, one hand pushing in and up, and then the other.

Rub Wrinkles Out: Cover face with warm hands, press face and pull hands away from nose out to ears, as if ironing or rubbing out wrinkles. Repeat.

Thumb Focus: Extend arm in front of you, with thumb up. Focus on the thumbnail, then change your depth of focus and concentrate on the wall or some far location behind the thumb. Go back and forth between the thumbnail and far away point, to sharpen your ability to change focus and depth perception. Repeat with other hand.

Head Rolling: Place top of head on flat surface of desk, palms flat on desktop. Roll the head around, releasing the stress and pain. If prefer, stand up and roll the head on the desktop.

Meditation: Rub hands together and place warm hands on eyes, fingers pointed up. Enjoy this energizing hideout for a moment or two. Repeat throughout the day, as needed.

HEMORRHOIDS: SEE CHAPTER 8 ON CONSTIPATION.

Seated Tree and Swaying Tree: lace the fingers and turn palms outward. Stretch the arms overhead, pulling in a giant breath. Exhale and bend at the waist to the right. Inhale as you come back up to center, exhale to the left. Repeat up to five times.

Seated Twist: Sit upright. Reach right arm across chest and reach behind left shoulder to hold back of chair, sliding hand along back of chair as far to right as possible. Keep fanny on seat. Turn head and look over right shoulder and continue to breathe. Take two complete breaths. Reverse, using left arm. Repeat up to five times on each side.

Seated Forward Bend: Sit with legs straight out in front, knees not bent, toes pointed upwards. Reaching out of the hips and shoulders, inhale deeply as you reach up high. On the slow exhale reach out in front of you (not collapsing) toward toes. Grab toes, ankles, shins or any part of legs you can comfortably reach. Breathe comfortably, letting the leg muscles stretch. Relax your back. Drop forehead to knees. Hold breath for five seconds. Return to starting position, do as many as comfortable.

Neck Release: Drop head between legs and hang. Such inversions relieve the rectum from being the lowest part of the body, for the pooling of blood.

Rectum lock: Sit comfortably with eyes closed and relax. Observe your natural breath. Pull up rectum and hold. Repeat as comfortable.

Rectum pulsing: Tighten and squeeze rectum, pulling it up and holding without strain as long as comfortable. Continue, rhythmically tightening and releasing the rectum, and being conscious of not adding other parts of the body such as thighs, buttocks or stomach to pulsation. Do throughout the day, as much as comfortable. Increase speed of contractions as able.

Diet: Avoid heavy foods such as cheese, meat, fried or oily dishes, and rich desserts. Enjoy soft, easily digestible foods such as fruit and vegetables.

HIPS

Hip disorders are one of the fastest growing afflictions of senior citizens in the West. Costly and often risky hip replacement surgeries are the last resort! Yoga and simple changes in how we sit can maintain our hip health and help us move gracefully into the next phase of our lives. In Ayurveda, we are taught a healthy hip is the key to longevity.

Eastern seniors have far, far fewer hip disorders (and back disorders) because they routinely sit cross-legged, opening up the hips, and on the floor, without a chair to weaken the back's natural support.

Half Butterfly: Bring right foot up and place on left thigh, as close to hip as able. Sit like this as long as comfortable, working at your desk or watching television. With right hand, lift right knee up and push back down to further stimulate the hip and release the synovial fluid lubricant (simulates one butterfly wing flapping!). Lift left heel off floor to increase the stretch. When ready, switch legs and repeat. Do often throughout the day. Finish with a nice full extension of each leg.

Rock the Twins: Bring right foot up and place on opposite knee. Lift up right leg, cradling like a baby from knee to foot, and rock side-to-side, loosening up hip. Switch legs.

Hip Circles: Pull left leg up to chest and lace hands around knee. Imagine your left thighbone is a large wooden spoon, and your buttock is a pot of chili on the stove. Your intention is to stir just the bottom of the chili pot. Slowly and subtly stir the chili, circling clockwise and counterclockwise, a small-refined circle. If you notice your foot is circling, you aren't stirring the pot. Focus on the hip joint only. Switch legs, repeat on right side.

Diet: Avoid meat. Excess protein settles in the joints. Drop extra pounds; stop asking our hips to carry more weight than their design allows.

Meditation: Sit quietly and comfortably, and reflect with honesty about how you would like to be more active in your life. Picture yourself with someone young (a grandchild, friend, puppy) and being able to play with them. See yourself enjoying rides at the County Fair. Commit yourself to having healthy hips.

IMMUNITY, ENDING THE MALAISE

Shining Skull: Close eyes and mouth, breathe only through nose. Take a few deep breaths to prepare. As you exhale, imagine you are snuffing a fly off your nose. The forced exhale feels like a short burst of breath, causing your abdominal muscles to contract briefly and your diaphragm to move down. Optionally, place your hands on belly, and feel your stomach pumping or jumping quickly. No inhale action required; this is called passive breathing. Repeat snuffing and pumping, one exhale per second. Start with three rounds of 20 to 30 pumpings. Gradually increase to 60 pumpings, one minute.

Alternate Nostril Breathing: Hold right hand up to nose, with elbow slightly tucked to your side and shoulder relaxed. Left hand resting on thigh. Gently close right nostril with right thumb and inhale from the left. Close left nostril with ring finger and exhale from right. Keep left nostril closed and inhale from right. Close right nostril with thumb and exhale from left. These steps comprise one round. Retention of breath can be added between each inhale and exhale, to promote the development of muscle mass.

Cross Your Heart: Close eyes. Cross arms at chest, placing palms under armpits. Press web between thumb and index finger deeply into crease of armpit, find the tender spot. Breathe deeply and slowly. Place other arm on top, repeat.

Squeeze and Tremble: Clasp hands together with arms partially extended directly in front of the chest, elbows slightly bent. Inhale as you squeeze hands together, pressing palms together as well as the space between fingers. It is normal to feel a tremble. Repeat five to eight times, wait 5 or 10 minutes and repeat indefinitely.

Energizer: Find center point between wrist and elbow and press down on inside of right arm. Locate center point on right side of top portion of arm, push down in center, between shoulder and elbow. Repeat on left arm.

Press and Roll: With palm facing up, use other hand to press the ends of each finger with thumb, rolling down from top of finger to first crease on finger. Flip hand over and do same procedure. Repeat on other hand. Like pressing a tube of toothpaste. Blood changes direction and returns to the heart at the tips of fingers and toes, so we regulate and activate the blood and blood pressure by squeezing tips.

Perineum Lock: Bring your attention to the point in front of your rectum, the perineum. Pull up this area to strengthen. Also helps with bladder weakness, incontinence. Can also be done lying down.

Special Practice: With fingertips of right hand, thump on the center of the breast bone, which is over the thymus gland. This gland, centered in what is known as the heart *chakra*, is known to be involved with immunity. Traditional medicine has taught that after one reaches age 25, the thymus is no longer active. Such thinking is no longer as certain, and many healers believe the gland can be stimulated into action with simple thumping.

Meditation: Fall in love with the word ―no.‖ Say ―no‖ to all invitations and offers that you honestly don't want to accept. Stop saying ―yes‖ when your body says ―no.‖ Enjoy being honest and your own company. Save your energy for what you truly care about. Please yourself first from now on. *Diet*: To maintain optimum health, eat a fresh plant diet (fruits, vegetables, grains and beans), loaded with vitamins, minerals, phytochemicals, antioxidants and carotenoids, all immunity-boosting compounds.

INCONTINENCE OF BLADDER, KIDNEY PROBLEMS, UTIS (URINARY TRACT INFECTIONS)

Bellows Breath: Two minutes of amplified, normal nose breathing. If you want to draw energy from above, imagine your breath is following a garland from your crown *chakra* down the front of the body through every *chakra*. At the root *chakra*, you begin to exhale up the garland on the back of the body, ending at the crown and begin again. If you wish to draw energy from the earth, begin the inhale at the root *chakra*, coming up to crown, with exhale going down back to root *chakra* and begin again. This breath can be gradually speeded up, and the length of time increased from two minutes, to fan the heat or fire.

Seated Forward Bend: sit with legs straight out in front, knees not bent, toes pointed upwards. Reaching out of the hips and shoulders, inhale deeply as you reach up high. On the slow exhale reach out in front of you, not collapsing, toward toes. Grab toes, ankles, shins or any part of legs you can comfortably reach. Breathe comfortably, letting the leg muscles stretch. Relax your back. Drop forehead to knees. Hold breath for five seconds. Return to starting position, do as many as comfortable.

Special Practice: Sitting on toilet, before passing anything, pour about two mugs of room temperature water on navel. Let water flow down into toilet, then urinate. Cools this overheated part of the body and helps strengthen continence. For UTIs, drink 1 tablespoon of apple cider vinegar in 8 ounces of room temperature water once or twice a day, for prevention and cure.

INDIGESTION

Everything starts with the digestion. Other than an accident or other external injury, most problems the body faces are due to bad digestion, and accompanying constipation. *See Chapter 8 on Constipation for in depth discussion.*

We all have a vulnerable or weak point due to our improper diet and subsequent bad digestion. If we eat too much of anything, even if it is pure ghee, it will cause an upset stomach and belching. When indigestion strikes, it is best to skip a meal and get the stomach clean.

When eating, particularly in a foreign country, if the bowel movement smells like the food you ate, then you aren't digesting properly. In such cases, you may well lack an enzyme, because you didn't grow up eating this kind of food. Try adding something that you easily digest, such as bread or toast, if you grew up on a wheat based diet, with the meal and see if digestion improves.

If bowel movement floats in toilet, this means you have absorbed all the nutrients in the food.

For acidity, *Alternate Nostril Breathing:* Hold right hand up to nose, with elbow slightly tucked to your side and shoulder relaxed. Left hand resting on thigh. Gently close right nostril with right thumb and inhale from the left. Close left nostril with ring finger and exhale from right. Keep left nostril closed and inhale from right. Close right nostril with thumb and exhale from left. These steps comprise one round. Retention of breath can be added between each inhale and exhale, to promote the development of muscle mass.

Humming Bee Breath: Three fingers placed not pressed on eyeballs, thumbs in ears. Inhale. On the exhale say *Om*, with five percent of the exhaled sound *O* of the *Om* and 95 percent of the exhaled sound the *M*. Concentrate on third eye and crown *chakra*. Sounds like a powerful bee has taken over the inside of the head. India's black bees are gigantic, patent leather doll shoes hovering over the mango flowers. As a Westerner, I think the Humming Bee sounds more like an 18-wheeler truck blasting its horn to warn of a head on collision.

Furnace Breath: Inhale making soft snoring noise in throat, like a baby sleeping. Swallow to hold breath. Exhale from left nostril only, holding right closed with right thumb. Do eight complete cycles. Removes phlegm from the throat and improves digestion.

Bellows Breath: Two minutes of amplified, normal nose breathing. If you want to draw energy from above, imagine your breath is following a garland from your crown *chakra* down the front of the body through every *chakra*. At the root *chakra*, you begin to exhale up the garland on the back of the body, ending at the crown and begin again. If you wish to draw energy from the earth, begin the inhale at the root *chakra*, coming up to crown, with exhale going down back to root *chakra* and begin again. This breath can be gradually speeded up, and the length of time increased from two minutes, to fan the heat or fire.

Fire Essence Breath: Exhale and tuck chin against neck/chest in chin lock. Rapidly pump the belly inside, contracting and expanding abdominal muscles. Try three rounds of 10 pumpings per round, to start. Inhale and exhale after each round. Build up to 60-100 pumpings per round. Cleans up digestive orders, constipation, strengthens abdomen. Best with empty stomach and bowels. *Do not do if more than three months pregnant.* Excellent after delivery, to tighten up pelvic and abdominal muscles. Proven to help flatten the abdomen.

Shining Skull: Close eyes and mouth, breathe only through nose. Take a few deep breaths to prepare. As you exhale, imagine you are snuffing a fly off your nose. The forced exhale feels like a short burst of breath, causing your abdominal muscles to contract briefly and your diaphragm to move down. Optionally, place your hands on belly, and feel your stomach pumping or jumping quickly. No inhale action required; this is called passive breathing. Repeat snuffing and pumping, one exhale per second. Start with three rounds of 20 to 30 pumpings. Gradually increase to 60 pumpings, one minute. For chronic indigestion and gas.

INHERITED AILMENTS

Hereditary afflictions are best addressed with breathing exercises.

Ramdev believes if this generation focuses on good living, genetic problems can actually be wiped out for the next generation. For example, parents with certain afflictions, like asthma, high blood pressure, and inherited joint problems should practice disciplined breathing exercises as a family. Getting children started young with Yoga, the risks of experiencing inherited diseases will be reduced, Ramdev teaches. By controlling health challenges in our lifetime, he says they won't be passed on to the next generation.

INSOMNIA

Humming Bee Breath: Three fingers placed not pressed on eyeballs, thumbs in ears. Inhale. On the exhale say Om, with five percent of the exhaled sound O of the Om and 95 percent of the exhaled sound the M. Concentrate on third eye and crown *chakra*. Sounds like a powerful bee has taken over the inside of the head. India's black bees are gigantic, patent leather doll shoes hovering over the mango flowers. As a Westerner, I think the Humming Bee sounds more like an 18-wheeler truck blasting its horn to warn of a head on collision.

Furnace Breath: Inhale making soft snoring noise in throat, like a baby sleeping. Swallow to hold breath. Exhale from left nostril only, holding right closed with right thumb. Do eight complete cycles. Removes phlegm from the throat and improves digestion.

Toe to Top Light Warm Ups at opening of this chapter.

Seated camel: Sit upright in a low backed chair or on a stool. Reach behind you and sit on your hands, fingers pointed forward, palm down. Arch back, drop head back and open chest, leaning over back of chair. Inhale and exhale deeply and slowly.

Meditation: Concentrated Gazing. Stare at a candle or image about two to three feet away, without blinking. When the eyes tire, close eyes and continue to meditate on the image of the flame, burned into the brain. When that image disappears, resume staring at the candle. Whenever thoughts arise, return to the flame. A lavender scented candle will act as a mild sedative, too.

Comfortably in bed, lie on left side (lying on right side tends to energize not relax). Count down in mind from 100 to 1, then do alternate nostril breathing. Both are done with stomach pulled in.

Diet: Vegetarians require less sleep than meat eaters. Digesting meat takes energy, and therefore, more sleep. Don't eat after 6 p.m., or your body will keep up, digesting all night. Stay away from caffeine after 12 noon. Avoid sugar and alcohol at night, it races through your body and keeps you awake, after the initial drugging wears off.

KNEES

Alternate Nostril Breathing: Hold right hand up to nose, with elbow slightly tucked to your side and shoulder relaxed. Left hand resting on thigh. Gently close right nostril with right thumb and inhale from the left. Close left nostril with ring finger and exhale from right. Keep left nostril closed and inhale from right. Close right nostril with thumb and exhale from left. These steps comprise one round. Retention of breath can be added between each inhale and exhale, to promote the development of muscle mass.

Leg Lifting Series: Sit upright. 1. Lift up one bent leg as high as comfortable, and then the other. 2. Life left foot up and touch heel to right knee. Reverse and do with right heel to left knee. 3. Kick one foot out, then the other. 4. Alternately extend legs out in front, digging heels into floor. Repeat each set in the series five to eight times on each side.

Kneecap Contraction: stretch the legs out in front of you and support right leg with left underneath it. Inhale and retain the breath, tightening the muscles around the right knee, pulling the kneecap up toward the thigh. Hold for few counts, exhale and relax. Reverse sides and repeat with right leg underneath. Repeat five times on each leg.

Knee Crank: Sit comfortably, pull left knee up and lace hands underneath the left thigh, in the crease of the knee, holding the weight of the thigh. Make circles with the lower leg, inhaling on the circle up and exhale on the down. Straighten the leg as much as able when foot heads toward ceiling. The rest of the body remains still. Circle 10 times in each direction and switch legs.

These poses can be done on full stomach. Never attempt if knee pain results.

Meditation: Sit comfortably and massage knees, slow but

strong. Use both hands on one knee, working all over and under to stimulate circulation. After massaging both knees with both hands, switch and place one hand on each knee for ongoing gentle massage. With eyes closed, think about how rarely you have ever stopped to massage and appreciate your knees. Spend some time reflecting on the importance of your knees, for absorbing the unexpected roadblocks, speed bumps, obstacles and potholes in your journey. In Ayurveda, the knees represent the brain. Spend a moment observing your mental activity. Have you been over thinking or excessively dwelling on some issue or person? It is time to ease up and become more flexible and trusting of the flow of life? Yawn often.

MEMORY, CONCENTRATION

Bellows Breath: Two minutes of amplified, normal nose breathing. If you want to draw energy from above, imagine your breath is following a garland from your crown *chakra* down the front of the body through every *chakra*. At the root *chakra*, you begin to exhale up the garland on the back of the body, ending at the crown and begin again. If you wish to draw energy from the earth, begin the inhale at the root *chakra*, coming up to crown, with exhale going down back to root *chakra* and begin again. This breath can be gradually speeded up, and the length of time increased from two minutes, to fan the heat or fire.

Blood to Brain: Open legs widely. Hang head and hands down with hands touching floor or as close as possible. Lift up heels so you are standing on toes, and lift heels up and down.

Special Practice: Place thumbs behind ears and rub down around ear, along edge of jaw and down on either side of windpipe. Repeat, always going one direction only, down. Pull and massage ears.

Meditation: Swami Rama teaches us that when we are interested in something, we give it attention and we remember it. If we wish to develop our memory, we must relax and take a real interest in the person or subject at hand. We remember who and what interests us.

Seated comfortably with eyes closed, begin to breathe deeply and rhythmically, silently counting from 1 to 100 and 100 to 1. Watch how many times your mind wanders and gets distracted. You must train your mind. Build upon this exercise, until you can count to and from 1000. Faithfully practicing this exercise sharpens the mind and creates a powerful ability to remember.

MENSTRUAL CRAMPS, PMS, MENOPAUSE, AND UTERINE FIBROIDS

Humming Bee Breath: Three fingers placed not pressed on eyeballs, thumbs in ears. Inhale. On the exhale say *Om*, with five percent of the exhaled sound *O* of the *Om* and 95 percent of the exhaled sound the *M*. Concentrate on third eye and crown *chakra*. Sounds like a powerful bee has taken over the inside of the head. India's black bees are gigantic, patent leather doll shoes hovering over the mango flowers. As a Westerner, I think the Humming Bee sounds more like an 18-wheeler truck blasting its horn to warn of a head on collision.

Alternate Nostril Breathing: Hold right hand up to nose, with elbow slightly tucked to your side and shoulder relaxed. Left hand resting on thigh. Gently close right nostril with right thumb and inhale from the left. Close left nostril with ring finger and exhale from right. Keep left nostril closed and inhale from right. Close right nostril with thumb and exhale from left. These steps comprise one round. Retention of breath can be added between each inhale and exhale, to promote the development of muscle mass.

Furnace Breath: Inhale making soft snoring noise in throat, like a baby sleeping. Swallow to hold breath. Exhale from left nostril only, holding right closed with right thumb. Do eight complete cycles. Removes phlegm from the throat and improves digestion.

Seated Forward Bend: sit with legs straight out in front, knees not bent, toes pointed upwards. Reaching out of the hips and shoulders, inhale deeply as you stretch high. On the slow exhale, reach out in front of you (not collapsing) toward toes. Grab toes, ankles, shins or any part of legs you can comfortably reach. Breathe comfortably, letting the leg muscles stretch. Relax your back. Drop forehead to knees. Hold breath for five seconds. Return to starting position, do as many as comfortable.

Seated Cat Stretch: Standing or sitting, place hands on thighs. Inhale, raise head and drop it back. Push the chest forward, humping the back. Hold a few seconds. Exhale while dropping chin to chest, pulling stomach in and squeezing all air out of body, arching back. Hold a few seconds. Do five to 10 rounds, with slow breath.

Knee Squeeze: Pull one knee at a time up to chest. Squeeze. Repeat four or more times with each leg. Then pull and hold both knees at chest.

Avoid inverted and strenuous poses when bleeding.

Rectum pulsing particularly helpful.

Diet: vegetarian with fresh fruit and salads, warm soothing beverages, especially catnip tea for cramping.

NECK

While modern medicine has developed some remarkable replacements for joints in the body, and in several cases, mastered the art of transplanting organs and other body parts, the neck is still irreplaceable.

Given its special and critical standing, we must treat it with great respect and gentleness.

Your neck spends most of the day holding up your 10 pound head. It is an incredibly versatile joint, the conduit for every message the brain sends. By regarding our neck as a junction or intersection, we quickly see the importance of keeping the pathways open, relaxed and flowing. Because it can move in so many ways, the neck symbolizes are ability to see many sides of a situation, far more than the old fashioned view of just two sides to every story. Without a neck that moves easily and freely, our ability to fully grasp a situation and remain open to different viewpoints is lost.

In our most primitive form, Homo sapiens knew that any threat to the neck was probably going to be fatal. Wild beasts, falling rocks and other natural disasters put the neck at great risk. As a consequence of this awareness, our conditioned response to any perceived danger, physical or emotional, involves tightening up the neck muscles.

In this millennium, wild humans are more likely the cause of our greatest tension. It is no accident that our language includes the well-worn phrase, —pain in the neck.‖ Individuals can definitely fit that definition, causing us to tighten up just at the mention of their name, let alone a sighting!

When we consider all the challenges faced every day in the workplace, highway and home, is it any surprise that most of us walk around with necks that resemble steel bridge cables?

A friend had been suffering severe, debilitating headaches for more than a year. His health insurance had been covering some astoundingly expensive MRIs, Cat Scans and other neurological tests, with no diagnosis forthcoming. Exploratory surgery of the cervical vertebrae was being discussed.

When I touched Al's neck, I was reminded of a granite pillar at the bank. —Have you had any massage?‖

—No,‖ Al joked, —My insurance won't cover it.

The end of the story is a happy one, remedied not by surgery but through massage and stretching. Getting away from the computer, the desk and television helps, too. One of the biggest culprits is the telephone; if you are still holding the handset by pinching up your shoulder and dropping your neck, stop! Go hands free, get a headset or use a speakerphone. Save yourself from chronic pain and surgery.

Furnace Breath: Inhale making soft snoring noise in throat, like a baby sleeping. Swallow to hold breath. Exhale from left nostril only, holding right closed with right thumb. Do eight complete cycles. Removes phlegm from the throat and improves digestion.

Neck Release: Close eyes. Sit upright, yet comfortable. Take a deep inhale and as you exhale, allow your hardworking neck to fall into your chest. Continue breathing, letting the neck hang. With every exhale, allow gravity to help your neck release more tightness, as you simply hang. Inhale and bring the head back to center, exhaling as you turn the head gently to the right. Breathe here for a few breaths. Inhale and on the exhale, turn the head gently to the left. Again, breathe here for a few moments. Inhale back to center, drop the head again on the exhale, hang and breathe. At your own pace, begin a series of slow circles with the neck, allowing yourself to release tension as you roll the head around the front to the back. Reverse directions and always make sure you are breathing. Do a few rounds and enjoy the release.

Arm Cradle: Drape right arm over head and touch left ear. Place left hand on left shoulder. Inhale fully, right up into the upper lobes of the lungs. On the exhale, gently let the head fall to the right, as both elbows drop down more toward the sides. All of your focus is on the space between the two hands...allow it to open and stretch. Stay here for a few breaths. Switch to the other side and repeat process.

Lap Cradle: Collapse into your lap, cradling your head in your knees. Put hands out, as if diving, then let them drop to your sides or hug your thighs. Breathe and relax. With each exhale, allow your neck to release. If your head does not reach your thighs comfortably, put a pillow in your lap.

Variation of lap cradle, lace fingers and place on the back of neck or head.

Hand Cradle: Place elbows on thighs and hold head in hands. Turn head in different positions, holding chin with one hand, ear with other. Hold chin and then forehead in hands.

Vertical Handshake: Place right hand on center back, elbow will be pointing upwards. Take left hand and bring behind back, reaching up toward right hand. Grasp shirt if needed (or have each hand hold the end of a towel, scarf or belt) and climb toward one another. See if you can shake hands. Upper elbow is ideally directly behind the head. For more of a challenge, look up. Reverse hands, placing left hand at top. Variation: Place right hand on center back. Take left hand and push right elbow down, stretching shoulder. Reverse hands.

Seated Twist: Sit upright. Take right arm and cross chest and reach behind shoulder to hold back of chair, sliding hand as far to right as possible. Keep fanny on seat. Turn head and look over right shoulder and continue to breathe. Take two complete breaths. Reverse, using left arm. Repeat up to five times.

Hand versus Head: Push right hand against side of head above ear, using resistance, inhaling through nose. Exhale. Place right hand at back of head, keep elbow out wide, inhale and push hand

and head with resistance. Exhale. Repeat on other side of head with left hand. With palms close together, hold chin with thumb and forefinger and on the inhale push hands into chin and resist with chin pushing back. Repeat full series five times.

Meditation: Sit or lie down comfortably. (If lying down, avoid pillow and lie on belly or back, with head centered, not turned to left or right.) Close eyes and tune into your natural breath. Imagine you are listening for a far away sound, like a puppy wanting to hear his master's car coming up the driveway. Cock your head this way and that, trying to catch the distant noise. Let your ear direct your neck.

Return to center and imagine you have a pencil taped to the end of your nose. Draw circles, from small to large, with your pencil, both directions. Try and sign your name with your nose! Yawn.

With all of this accomplished, breathe comfortably, if you are sitting, allow your head to hang. Think of being the wise old owl, able to survey an entire scene with a flexible neck.

PARALYSIS AND STROKE

Though the link might not appear direct, in the East it is believed paralysis is ultimately caused by constipation. *See Chapter 8 on Constipation. Follow the same program as for high blood pressure. Waste and fat strangle the veins.*

All Breathing exercises done in a gentle fashion are helpful, especially:

Alternate Nostril Breathing: Hold right hand up to nose, with elbow slightly tucked to your side and shoulder relaxed. Left hand resting on thigh. Gently close right nostril with right thumb and inhale from the left. Close left nostril with ring finger and exhale from right. Keep left nostril closed and inhale from right. Close right nostril with thumb and exhale from left. These steps comprise one round. Retention of breath can be added between each inhale and exhale, to promote the development of muscle mass.

Humming Bee Breath: Three fingers placed not pressed on eyeballs, thumbs in ears. Inhale. On the exhale say *Om*, with five percent of the exhaled sound *O* of the *Om* and 95 percent of the exhaled sound the *M*. Concentrate on third eye and crown *chakra*. Sounds like a powerful bee has taken over the inside of the head. India's black bees are gigantic, patent leather doll shoes hovering over the mango flowers. As a Westerner, I think the Humming Bee sounds more like an 18-wheeler truck blasting its horn to warn of a head on collision.

Furnace Breath: Inhale making soft snoring noise in throat, like a baby sleeping. Swallow to hold breath. Exhale from left nostril only, holding right closed with right thumb. Do eight complete cycles. Removes phlegm from the throat and improves digestion.

Squeeze and Tremble: Clasp hands together with arms partially extended directly in front of the chest, elbows slightly bent. Inhale as you squeeze hands together, pressing palms together as well as the space between fingers. It is normal to feel a tremble. Repeat five to eight times, wait five or 10 minutes and repeat indefinitely.

PEPTIC ULCER

Rolled Pipe Tongue Cooling Breath: Roll tongue like a pipe, stick out of mouth and inhale, drawing air over tongue. If you can't roll your tongue, this is actually an inherited talent, do the *Hissing Breath*: Slightly open mouth, with teeth slightly parted and tongue planted behind lower teeth and inhale. For both styles of cooling breath, after inhaling, swallow and exhale through left nostril, holding right nostril closed with right thumb. Repeat five-eight times.

Only one pose is good after eating to aid digestion: sit on haunches with hands upon thighs or hanging down at sides, and breathe deeply.

Wrist Knead: Rub wrists with other hand. Using four fingertips in a row perpendicular to femur, knead up to four inches from wrist. This attention massages all the nadis or channels of the digestion system, and the practice is like giving one's inner organs a massage.

Diet: Eat a small bit of apple, the size of a small walnut with your meal. As much as a quarter of an apple can be eaten while eating other foods. Adding cinnamon to warm drink or porridge encourages digestion, treats gas. To not produce gas, chew food slowly, avoid gulping air. Limit bean intake.

Meditation: For food allergies or intolerances, rather than mourn what you miss, find pleasure in knowing that the foods you can't eat are for someone else to eat and enjoy. Be glad for others.

POSTURE

Alternate Nostril Breathing: Hold right hand up to nose, with elbow slightly tucked to your side and shoulder relaxed. Left hand resting on thigh. Gently close right nostril with right thumb and inhale from the left. Close left nostril with ring finger and exhale from right. Keep left nostril closed and inhale from right. Close right nostril with thumb and exhale from left. These steps comprise one round. Retention of breath can be added between each inhale and exhale, to promote the development of muscle mass.

Pray Behind Your Back: Sit upright, away from back of chair. Bring hands behind back; bring fingertips together, pointing up. If able, bring hands together in prayer and move up the spine.

Hold and Release Beach Ball: Imagine you are holding a giant beach ball, so large it makes your chest cave in to hold it. Exhale fully to better get a hold of the ball. Suddenly, take a great inhale and pull your outstretched arms back as far as you can, puffing up the chest and letting the ball go. Repeat up to five times.

Hand versus Head: Push right hand against side of head above ear, using resistance, inhaling through nose. Exhale. Place right hand at back of head, keep elbow out wide, inhale and push hand and head with resistance. Exhale. Repeat on other side of head with left hand. With palms close together, hold chin with thumb and forefinger and on the inhale push hands into chin and resist with chin pushing back. Repeat full series five times.

Airplane Propeller: Lock fingers together at chest level with elbows bent straight out to either side. Inhale and point the right elbow toward the ceiling. Exhale and send the left elbow up to the ceiling. Continue to move your propeller with your breath, opening up the chest and shoulders.

Vertical Handshake: Place right hand on center back, elbow will be pointing upwards. Take left hand and bring behind back, reaching up toward right hand. Grasp shirt if needed (or have each hand hold the end of a towel, scarf or belt) and climb toward one another. See if you can shake hands. Upper elbow is ideally directly behind the head. For more of a challenge, look up. Reverse hands, placing left hand at top. Variation: Place right hand on center back. Take left hand and push right elbow down, stretching shoulder. Reverse hands.

Do poses listed in Shoulder section.

Meditation: Your posture is as revealing as your face in telling your life story. As the eyes are the windows of the soul, your weak or strong back provides plenty of information about how you are living your life.

Women who are either self conscious about their height or breasts learn at an early age to roll their shoulders forward and pull in the chest. Tall men also can dip down or send the neck and head way out in front of them, in an effort to make closer eye contact with shorter people.

Often, feeling beaten down by the trials of daily routines, our backs can begin to mirror or reflect this air of resignation. Shoulders slump forward and down, the back curves. Our lungs are compromised, as the front of the body also sinks in and down, crushing the organs of digestion.

Rather than greeting the world with a strong back and a soft approachable front, we subconsciously reverse these energies. In our despair, we present a hardened or toughened front and a weak, unsupportive spine. The world is no longer our home where we trust and reach out, but the place we feel victimized and overwhelmed. The message others receive is something like, —Feels like a loser. Needs a lot of propping up from others. Hazardous to your health; avoid!‖

Examine your posture. Avoid the temptation to overcorrect and become ramrod straight like the metal-displaying five star general, ready for battle. Adopting this armed and dangerous stance, you will be just as off-putting and unappealing as when in the loser posture. Rather, find that balance between hopelessness and intimidation. What you seek is to be upstanding in your own life, with a tender open front and a strong back to carry you.

Just the way you stand and sit can determine the quality of

your day and your relationships. Close your eyes and mouth. Sit comfortably, back straight, feet on the floor. Breathing through the nose, allow your lungs to fully fill and empty. Find and hold your natural healthy posture and begin to live from this place.

PREGNANCY

To prepare for delivery, do lots of walking, no jumping.

Furnace Breath: Inhale making soft snoring noise in throat, like a baby sleeping. Swallow to hold breath. Exhale from left nostril only, holding right closed with right thumb. Do eight complete cycles. Removes phlegm from the throat and improves digestion.

Humming Bee Breath: Three fingers placed not pressed on eyeballs, thumbs in ears. Inhale. On the exhale say *Om*, with five percent of the exhaled sound *O* of the *Om* and 95 percent of the exhaled sound the *M*. Concentrate on third eye and crown *chakra*. Sounds like a powerful bee has taken over the inside of the head. India's black bees are gigantic, patent leather doll shoes hovering over the mango flowers. As a Westerner, I think the Humming Bee sounds more like an 18-wheeler truck blasting its horn to warn of a head on collision.

Clock Face: Imagine your face is a clock. Think of random hours, and look at the appropriate area of your face. For example, three o'clock is directly to your right, and 12 is straight up. Move only your eyes. Go in both directions, diagonally and other ways. Breathe slowly and deeply. Strengthens eyes and restores roundness to eyeball. Preferable to do with eyes open.

Thumb Focus: Extend arm in front of you, with thumb up. Focus on the thumbnail, then change your depth of focus and concentrate on the wall or some far location behind the thumb. Go back and forth between the thumbnail and far away point, to sharpen your ability to change focus and depth perception. Repeat with other hand.

Rock the Twins: Bring right foot up and place on opposite knee. Lift up right leg, cradling like a baby from knee to foot, and rock side-to-side, loosening up hip. Switch legs.

Seated Twist: Sit upright. Reach right arm across chest and reach behind left shoulder to hold back of chair, sliding hand along back of chair as far to right as possible. Keep fanny on seat. Turn head and look over right shoulder and continue to breathe. Take two complete breaths. Reverse, using left arm. Repeat up to five times on each side

Seated Tree and Swaying Tree: Lace fingers in front of body and turn palms outward. Stretch the arms overhead, pulling in a giant breath. Exhale and bend at the waist to the right. Inhale as you come back up to center, exhale to the left. Repeat up to five times, each side.

In labor, do *Alternate Nostril Breathing:* Hold right hand up to nose, with elbow slightly tucked to your side and shoulder relaxed. Left hand resting on thigh. Gently close right nostril with right thumb and inhale from the left. Close left nostril with ring finger and exhale from right. Keep left nostril closed and inhale from right. Close right nostril with thumb and exhale from left. These steps comprise one round.

After delivery, new mothers in India are told the best way to restore vitality is to do no real exercise for three months.

PROSTATE HEALTH

Sit upright. Close eyes. Inhale slowly and fully, hold breath. Pull up/tighten/contract pelvic floor, the perineum-rectal area. Hold until need to exhale. Release lock and then inhale. Tones the system of elimination, helps with relieving constipation and hemorrhoids. Good for chronic pelvic and prostate infections.

SCIATICA

Seated camel: Sit upright in a low backed chair or on a stool. Reach behind you and sit on your hands, fingers pointed forward, palm down. Arch back, drop head back and open chest, leaning over back of chair. Inhale and exhale deeply and slowly.

Knee Squeeze: Pull one knee at a time up to chest. Squeeze. Repeat four or more times with each leg. Then pull and hold both knees at chest.

Bent Leg Lifts: Place right foot on left knee. Lace hands around left knee and pull knee toward chest as close as possible. Reverse, do opposite leg. Also called the pyriformis squeeze.

SHOULDERS

Alternate Nostril Breathing: Hold right hand up to nose, with elbow slightly tucked to your side and shoulder relaxed. Left hand resting on thigh. Gently close right nostril with right thumb and inhale from the left. Close left nostril with ring finger and exhale from right. Keep left nostril closed and inhale from right. Close right nostril with thumb and exhale from left. These steps comprise one round.

Psychic Union: Sit and close eyes. Lace hands behind back. Inhale deeply. When exhaling, fall forward, spine straight, bringing forehead as close to lap as possible, arms up behind you. Stay and breathe as long as comfortable. Relax into stretch, let gravity help you to fall even further down, lifting arms above you.

Back and Forth: Sit straight, reach back with both arms and grab back of chair. Keep holding chair and lean back, stretches pectorals and upper arms, then lean forward over knees, continuing to hold back of chair. Pulse back and forth in small movement.

Seated Tree and Swaying: Lace fingers in front of body and turn palms outward. Stretch the arms overhead, pulling in a giant breath. Exhale and bend at the waist to the right. Inhale as you come back up to center, exhale to the left. Repeat up to five times, each side.

Vertical Handshake: Place right hand on center back, elbow will be pointing upwards. Take left hand and bring behind back, reaching up toward right hand. Grasp shirt if needed (or have each hand hold the end of a towel, scarf or belt) and climb toward one another. See if you can shake hands. Upper elbow is ideally directly behind the head. For more of a challenge, look up. Reverse hands, placing left hand at top. Variation: Place right hand on center back. Take left hand and push right elbow down, stretching shoulder. Reverse hands.

Get Off My Back: Place clenched fist at bottom of ribcage. Lift elbows as high as you can at your sides, up behind you. Swing fists forward and back, adding the audio, —get off my back‖ in staccato bursts with your breath, each time you pull the elbows back. Feel the release.

Turtle in the Shell, Swan Neck: On inhale pull the shoulders up to the ears. Hold. On exhale, drop shoulders down as far as possibly, lengthening neck, like swan.

Wing Circles: Close eyes. Place left hand on left shoulder, right hand on right shoulder. Circle your wings, work to bring elbows to touch each other in front. Reverse directions. Drop hands and circle shoulders in one direction and then the other, then circle the shoulders in opposite directions at the same time.

Rake and Shake: Place right hand near or above left shoulder blade. Support right elbow with left hand. Using right hand, look for pain in your shoulder blade area. Squeeze, poke, pinch, knead, rub. Use four strong fingers and rake from shoulder blade up over shoulder, then shake off the pain from your hand and repeat. Reverse sides and use left hand on right shoulder blade.

Pray Behind Your Back: Sit upright, away from back of chair. Bring hands behind back; bring fingertips together, pointing up. If able, bring hands together in prayer and move up the spine.

Hold and Release Beach Ball: Imagine you are holding a giant beach ball, so large it makes your chest cave in to hold it. Exhale fully to better get a hold of the ball. Suddenly, take a great inhale and pull your outstretched arms back as far as you can, puffing up the chest and letting the ball go. Repeat up to five times.

Triple Hug: Cross arms in front of chest, wrap hands around neck; try to lace fingers behind neck. Switch, put opposite hand on top and repeat. Go to shoulders, again with arms crossed, and reach hands around to touch opposite shoulder blade. Keep walking the fingers back to deepen the hug. Switch, put opposite hand on top and repeat. Go to your waist (remember it?) again with arms crossed, see if you can walk hands around toward back. Switch, put opposite hand on top and repeat.

Chopping Wood: Clasp hands together inhale and raise arms as high as possible above head and even behind head, stretching spine. Look up at hands. Make a strong down stroke with clasped hands on the exhale, emitting a —ha! sound. Repeat 5-10 times.

Ringing the Bell: Inhale and reach high about head with hands gripping imaginary rope. Exhale and pull the rope down with vigor, ringing the Liberty Bell. Repeat 5-10 times. Also firms breast, muscles of chest and stretches upper back.

Meditation: Tightness across the shoulder blades, shoulders seized up around the ears and general shoulder pain relate to the shouldering of responsibility. We can easily feel we are carrying the weight of the world on our shoulders and upper back. For some of us, it feels like we are hauling a grand piano around in our backpack. See the word *should* in shoulder; are you *shoulding* all over yourself?

Sit comfortably, with the eyes closed. Treat yourself to a few yawns. Breathing through the nose only, imagine your inhale is filling the entire chest and going into the shoulders. As you exhale, let go of the aches, pains and tension from the shoulders.

Inhale a soothing healing color, perhaps sunny yellow or pure brilliant white. Pull this color into the shoulders, letting it reach all the nooks and crannies where you have stored duty and pain. Exhale a color that denotes letting go of the old. See that which no longer serves you drift off on the smoke of your breath. Release all that is no longer serving you, unrealistic expectations, heavy memories, weighty decisions. Continue to sit and breathe, experiencing your lighter load.

SINUS

Bellows Breath: Two minutes of amplified, normal nose breathing. If you want to draw energy from above, imagine your breath is following a garland from your crown *chakra* down the front of the body through every *chakra*. At the root *chakra*, you begin to exhale up the garland on the back of the body, ending at the crown and begin again. If you wish to draw energy from the earth, begin the inhale at the root *chakra*, coming up to crown, with exhale going down back to root *chakra* and begin again. This breath can be gradually speeded up, and the length of time increased from two minutes, to fan the heat or fire.

Roaring Lion: Place your hands, fingers spread wide, on your thighs, like giant paws. Sit upright and inhale deeply. Lean forward, as if to pounce on your prey, stick your tongue out and down, roll your eyes up and exhale with a loud throaty roar! You're a lion, not a kitten, so don't hold back. Clears out the lungs and throat.

Repeat three times, or until you clear your throat and scare your prey.

Knee to Nose: Sit with feet on ground. Lift left leg up and touch knee to nose. Reverse, do other leg. Repeat.

Cross Your Heart: Sit with flat hands underneath opposite armpit. Squeeze point between thumb and first finger firmly and breathe. Eyes closed, breathe through nose only. For blocked nostrils, make fists with hands. Repeat up to 5-10 minutes, if needed.

Diet: First, have a good diet; remove all whites, all wheat, rice, ice cream, and dairy. Eat very little at night, especially if it is cold at night, don't eat any cold food.

Meditation: Before getting out of bed in the morning, YogaSir says touch the ground to worship the Earth, then bring your hands to face. According to India's ancient sacred scriptures, the *Vedas*, this effort has holy and enriching powers. The three sections of the hands (fingers and upper and lower palm) represent prosperity, education and health, so by touching the Earth in reverence, a blessing is received.

Again, before rising, check your nostrils to see which one is open and which one is blocked. Put fingers under nostrils, one at a time, to determine which one is not exhaling. If the right nostril is open, put your right foot first on the ground, then take three small steps to the right. If left is blocked, take your steps to the left, but take four. Within a short period, the sinus problem will be cured.

SKIN

All breathing exercises are appropriate.

Crossed Hands Raised: Tying the breath to the movement of the arms, begin with hands crossed hanging in front. Inhale and raise arms overhead, again crossing hands over the head. Drop head back to look up at hands. Exhale and bring arms out to sides, straight out from shoulders. Inhale back above head, crossed hands. Exhale swing arms down and hang crossed hands in front of body. Repeat entire cycle five to 10 times

Diet: Avoid fried and oily foods, spicy foods, sweets, non-vegetarian foods.

Meditation: the skin is our largest organ, sensory communicator and our greatest protector. Sit and experience the feeling of being safe and secure in your own skin, your natural barrier. Trust yourself and your feelings. Let go of any sense of being at risk or threatened, and the need to grow thick skin, a hide or shield. Love and thank your skin for being your first line of defense.

If skin problems are on the face, avoid any temptation to pick at skin, cuticle or nail on big toe, which represents the face.

THIRST AND HUNGER

Rolled Pipe Tongue Cooling Breath: Roll tongue like a pipe, stick out of mouth and inhale, drawing air over tongue. If you can't roll your tongue, this is actually an inherited talent, do the *Hissing Breath*: Slightly open mouth, with teeth slightly parted and tongue planted behind lower teeth and inhale. For both styles of cooling breath, after inhaling, swallow and exhale through left nostril, holding right nostril closed with right thumb. Repeat five-eight times. *To control hunger, see Weight Loss section and Chapter 7.*

THYROID

Furnace Breath: Inhale making soft snoring noise in throat, like a baby sleeping. Swallow to hold breath. Exhale from left nostril only, holding right closed with right thumb. Do eight complete cycles. Removes phlegm from the throat and improves digestion.

Bellows Breath: Two minutes of amplified, normal nose breathing. If you want to draw energy from above, imagine your breath is following a garland from your crown *chakra* down the front of the body through every *chakra*. At the root *chakra*, you begin to exhale up the garland on the back of the body, ending at the crown and begin again. If you wish to draw energy from the earth, begin the inhale at the root *chakra*, coming up to crown, with exhale going down back to root *chakra* and begin again. This breath can be gradually speeded up, and the length of time increased from two minutes, to fan the heat or fire.

Humming Bee Breath: Three fingers placed not pressed on eyeballs, thumbs in ears. Inhale. On the exhale say *Om*, with five percent of the exhaled sound *O* of the *Om* and 95 percent of the exhaled sound the *M*. Concentrate on third eye and crown *chakra*. Sounds like a powerful bee has taken over the inside of the head. India's black bees are gigantic, patent leather doll shoes hovering over the mango flowers. As a Westerner, I think the Humming Bee sounds more like an 18-wheeler truck blasting its horn to warn of a head on collision.

Toe to Top Light Warm Ups at opening of this chapter.

Neck Release with Chin Lock: Close eyes. Sit upright, yet comfortable. Take a deep inhale and as you exhale, allow your hardworking neck to fall into your chest. Continue breathing, letting the neck hang. With every exhale, allow gravity to help your neck release more tightness, as you simply hang. Lock down chin, squeezing into chest and neck. Inhale and bring the head back to center, exhaling as you turn the head gently to the right. Breathe here for a few breaths. Inhale. On the exhale, turn the head gently to the left. Again, breathe here for a few moments. Inhale back to center, drop the head again on the exhale, hang and breathe. At your own pace, begin a series of slow circles with the neck, allowing yourself to release tension as you roll the head around the front to the back. Reverse directions and always make sure you are breathing. Do a few rounds and enjoy the release.

Special Practice: Place thumbs behind ears and rub down around ear, along edge of jaw and down on either side of windpipe. Repeat, always going one direction only, down.

TONGUE

If a film appears on the tongue, incomplete digestion is the cause. Mouth cankers are frequently due to excessive sugar.

Rolled Pipe Tongue Cooling Breath: Roll tongue like a pipe, stick out of mouth and inhale, drawing air over tongue. If you can't roll your tongue, this is actually an inherited talent, do the *Hissing Breath*: Slightly open mouth, with teeth slightly parted and tongue planted behind lower teeth and inhale. For both styles of cooling breath, after inhaling, swallow and exhale through left nostril, holding right nostril closed with right thumb. Repeat five-eight times.

Cooling Moon Breath: With right hand, use thumb to close right nostril and ring finger to close left. Inhale through left and exhale through right, repeatedly. Useful during warm weather or when the body feels warm, as it is cooling.

Diet: Switch to a bland, simple diet for a few days to isolate the cause. Reduce intake of starches. Avoid all sugars and sweetened drinks, including alcohol.

Tonsil or Throat Ailments, Including Cough

Furnace Breath: Inhale making soft snoring noise in throat, like a baby sleeping. Swallow to hold breath. Exhale from left nostril only, holding right closed with right thumb. Do eight complete cycles. Removes phlegm from the throat and improves digestion.

Roaring Lion: Place your hands, fingers spread wide, on your thighs, like giant paws. Sit upright and inhale deeply. Lean forward, as if to pounce on your prey, stick your tongue out and down, roll your eyes up and exhale with a loud throaty roar! You're a lion, not a kitten, so don't hold back. Clears out the lungs and throat. Repeat three times, or until you clear your throat and scare your prey.

Special Practice: Place thumbs behind ears and rub down around ear, along edge of jaw and down on either side of windpipe. Repeat, always going one direction only, down.

Vertigo and Dizziness

Humming Bee Breath: Three fingers placed not pressed on eyeballs, thumbs in ears. Inhale. On the exhale say Om, with five percent of the exhaled sound O of the Om and 95 percent of the exhaled sound the M. Concentrate on third eye and crown *chakra*. Sounds like a powerful bee has taken over the inside of the head. India's black bees are gigantic, patent leather doll shoes hovering over the mango flowers. As a Westerner, I think the Humming Bee sounds more like an 18-wheeler truck blasting its horn to warn of a head on collision.

Improving inner balance is helpful. Practice standing with your eyes closed. Practice standing on one leg.

Meditation: Think about why you might be unconsciously choosing to be in a confused state now, rather than facing a situation that feels difficult. Perhaps you are approaching a decision that seems black and white, and you fear repercussions or ramifications? Expand your view of the circumstances, and look for new ways to relate. Become clear headed in your resolve to handle an unresolved matter.

WEIGHT—TO GAIN

Fire Essence Breath: Exhale and tuck chin against neck/chest in chin lock. Rapidly pump the belly inside, contracting and expanding abdominal muscles. Try three rounds of 10 pumpings per round, to start. Inhale and exhale after each round. Build up to 60-100 pumpings per round. Cleans up digestive orders, constipation, strengthens abdomen. Best with empty stomach and bowels. *Do not do if more than three months pregnant.* Excellent after delivery, to tighten up pelvic and abdominal muscles. Proven to help flatten the abdomen.

Alternate Nostril Breathing: Hold right hand up to nose, with elbow slightly tucked to your side and shoulder relaxed. Left hand resting on thigh. Gently close right nostril with right thumb and inhale from the left. Close left nostril with ring finger and exhale from right. Keep left nostril closed and inhale from right. Close right nostril with thumb and exhale from left. These steps comprise one round. Retention of breath can be added between each inhale and exhale, to promote the development of muscle mass.

When doing breathing exercises always add pause and be still, holding the breath, between inhale and exhale.

Seated Sun Salutation: Make sure you have plenty of room beside and behind you. Stand in front of your chair, facing the seat.

1. Raise hands overhead, inhale, stretching backwards are far as comfortable.

2. Exhale bend forward and grasp the sides of the chair or seat, bringing your head toward the seat. In traditional Sun Salutation, hands are on the floor here.

3. Holding on to chair, inhale and stretch right leg out behind you.

4. Stretch left leg out, as far back as comfortable.

5. Hold breath and posture (with both legs extended behind you) for a moment, this posture is called Plank.

6. Exhale, slightly lower chest and belly while body is extended, if possible.

7. Inhale raise chin up and tip head back, puffing out chest in seated Cobra.

8. Exhale; bring right leg back to front.

9. Inhale, bring left leg back up to front.

10. Exhale, let go of chair and let arms and head hang down.

11. Slowly raise arms up in big inhaling salutation

12. Exhale arms to sides.

Repeat steps, stretching left leg out first behind you in step 3 and then right. This is one complete Salutation. Start with doing one complete Salutation and build up.

WEIGHT—TO LOSE

Any and all breathing exercises, especially *Bellows Breath* to fire up digestion.

Bellows Breath: Two minutes of amplified, normal nose breathing. If you want to draw energy from above, imagine your breath is following a garland from your crown *chakra* down the front of the body through every *chakra*. At the root *chakra*, you begin to exhale up the garland on the back of the body, ending at the crown and begin again. If you wish to draw energy from the earth, begin the inhale at the root *chakra*, coming up to crown, with exhale going down back to root *chakra* and begin again. This breath can be gradually speeded up, and the length of time increased from two minutes, to fan the heat or fire.

Alternate Nostril Breathing: Hold right hand up to nose, with elbow slightly tucked to your side and shoulder relaxed. Left hand resting on thigh. Gently close right nostril with right thumb and inhale from the left. Close left nostril with ring finger and exhale from right. Keep left nostril closed and inhale from right. Close right nostril with thumb and exhale from left. These steps comprise one round.

Shining Skull: Close eyes and mouth, breathe only through nose. Take a few deep breaths to prepare. As you exhale, imagine you are snuffing a fly off your nose. The forced exhale feels like a short burst of breath, causing your abdominal muscles to contract briefly and your diaphragm to move down. Optionally, place your hands on belly, and feel your stomach pumping or jumping quickly. No inhale action required; this is called passive breathing. Repeat snuffing and pumping, one exhale per second. Start with three rounds of 20 to 30 pumpings. Gradually increase to 60 pumpings, one minute.

Do next three to satisfy cravings.

Rolled Pipe Tongue Cooling Breath: Roll tongue like a pipe, stick out of mouth and inhale, drawing air over tongue. If you can't roll your tongue, this is actually an inherited talent, do the *Hissing Breath*: Slightly open mouth, with teeth slightly parted and tongue planted behind lower teeth and inhale. For both styles of cooling breath, after inhaling, swallow and exhale through left nostril, holding right nostril closed with right thumb. Repeat five-eight times. Variation: Fold tongue back and suck air over tongue during inhale.

Do any and all Yoga poses vigorously! Focus on those with resistance. Lift self in seat, hands at side.

Locomotive Power: Sit upright, mouth closed, with elbows bent and arms pointing upward, palms near ears. Breathing through the nose only, shoot the arms forcefully up on the inhale. Making fists, exhaling forcefully through the nose only, pull the arms down quickly and forcefully. Repeat and rest. Build up to 50 locomotions, perhaps even breaking a sweat. Your locomotive burns calories.

Meditation: Discover why you are building a wall around you, why you feel unsafe and need to hide yourself and/or your shape. Look at why you are eating someone else's share. In your mind's eye, observe yourself eating sweets, observe your need for something sweet and lovely in your life, something that is not edible.

BIBLIOGRAPHY

Ajaya, Swami, <u>Psychotherapy East and West: A Unifying Paradigm</u>, The Himalayan International Institute of Yoga Science and Philosophy, Honesdale, PA, 1997

Anderson, Norman B., <u>Emotional Longevity: What Really Determines How Long You Live,</u> Viking, NY, NY, 2003

Bahm, A. J., <u>Yoga Sutras of Patanjali</u>, Asian Humanities Press, Berkeley, CA, 1993

Byrd, Richard E., <u>Alone: The Classic Polar Adventure</u>, Shearwater Book, Island Press, Washington, DC, 2003

Caplin, Joan, —Mobilizing the Compromised Immune System in Catastrophic Illness Interview with Lawrence LeShan, Ph.D.‖, Consumer News, Vol. 1, No. 8, August 1996

Carter, Mildred, <u>Body Reflexology: Healing at your Fingertips</u>, Parker Publishing Co., 1994 (any book by Carter is good)

Coulter, H. David, <u>Anatomy of Yoga</u>, Body and Breath, Inc., Honesdale, PA, 2001

Davies, Clair, <u>The Trigger Point Therapy Workbook: Your Self-Treatment Guide for Pain Relief,</u> New Harbinger Publications, Oakland, CA, 2001

Day, Harvey <u>Executive Yoga: A Practical System for the Busy Man</u>, Pinnacle Books, NY, NY, 1972

Folan, Lilias,<u> Lilias Yoga and You</u>, Bantam Books, NY, NY, 1976

Gach, Michael Reed, <u>The Acupressure Stress Management Book: Acu-Yoga</u>, Japan Publications, Inc., Tokyo, 1981

Grout, Pam, <u>Jumpstart Your Metabolism, How to Lose Weight by Changing the Way You Breathe</u>, A Fireside Book, Simon and Schuster, NY, NY, 1998

Hanh, Thich Nhat, <u>Being Peace</u>, Parallax Press, 2005

Hart, William, <u>The Art of Living: Vipassana Meditation</u>, Vipassana Research Institute, Maharashtra, India, 2005

Hansard, Christopher, The Tibetan Art of Living, Atria Books, NY, NY, 2001

Hay, Louise, Heal Your Body A to Z, the Mental Causes for Physical Illness and the Metaphysical Way to Overcome Them, Hay House Publishing, Carlsbad, CA, 1982

Hendler, Sheldon Saul, The Oxygen Breath through,
Random House Value Publishing, NY, NY, 1991

Hittleman, Richard, Introduction to Yoga, Bantam Books, NY,NY, 1980

Hosseini, Khaled, The Kite Runner, Penguin Books, 2004

Levine, Barbara Hoberan, Your Body Believes Every Word You Say, Aslan Publishing, Lower Lake, CA, 1991

Hay, Louise L, Gratitude: A Way of Life, Hay House Publications, Oakland, CA, 1996

Hendler, Sheldon Saul, The Oxygen Breakthrough: 30 Days To an Illness Free Life, William Morrow & Co, 1989

Ibid, Heal Your Body: The Mental Causes for Physical Illness and the Metaphysical Way to Overcome Them, Hay House Publications, Oakland, CA, 2005

Ibid, You Can Heal Your Life, Hay House Publications, Oakland, CA, 2004

Kroeger, Hanna, The Basic Causes of Modern Diseases and How to Remedy Them, Hay House Publications, Carlsbad, CA, 1998

LeShan, Lawrence, Cancer As a Turning Point: A Handbook for People with Cancer, Their Families, and Health Professionals, Plume, Penguin Group, NY, NY, 1994

Maharaj, Sri Nisargadatta, I Am That, Kavi Arya Press, Bombay, 1999

Main OSB, John, "All You Have to Do is Begin," Word Made Flesh, London: Darton, Longman, 1993

Mate, Gabor, When the Body Says No: Understanding the Stress – Disease Connection, John Wiley and Sons, Inc., Hoboken, NJ, 2003

Pennington, Basil, Centering Prayer: Renewing an Ancient Christian Prayer Form, Image Books, Doubleday, NY, NY, 1982

Pierce, Margaret D. and Martin G., Yoga for your Life, Sterling Publishing Company, NY, NY, 1996

Editors of Prevention Magazine, <u>Hands-on Healing: Massage Remedies for Hundreds of Health Problems,</u> Rodale Press, Inc, Emmaus, PA, 1989

Prudden, Bonnie, <u>How to Keep Your Family Fit and Healthy</u>, Reader's Digest Press; distributed by E. P. Dutton, NY, NY, 1975

Rama, Swami, <u>The Art of Joyful Living</u>, Himalayan Institute Press, Honesdale, PA, Fusion Books, New Delhi, 2004

Rama, Swami, <u>Meditation and Its Practice</u>, Himalayan Institute Press, Honesdale, PA, 1998

Rama, Swami, <u>Perennial Psychology of the Bhagavad-Gita</u>, The Himalayan International Institute of Yoga Science and Philosophy of the USA, Honesdale, PA, Fusion Books, New Delhi, 2004

Saraswati, Swami Satyananda, <u>Asana Pranayama Mudra Bandha</u>, Bihar School of Yoga, Munger, Bihar, India, 1999

Selby, John, <u>Seven Masters, One Path: Meditation Secrets from the World's Greatest Masters,</u> Harper One, 2003

Sinclair, Upton, <u>The Jungle</u>, University of Illinois Press, Champaign, IL, 1988.

Sivananda, Swami, <u>The Bhagavad-Gita: Word to Word Meaning, Translation and Commentary,</u> Divine Life Society Tehr-Garhwal, UP, India, 1995

Sivananda Yoga Center, <u>The Sivananda Companion to Yoga</u>, A Fireside Book, Simon and Schuster, NY, NY, 2000

Sivananda Yoga Vendanta Centers, The Yoga Cookbook, A Fireside Book, Simon & Schuster, NY,NY 1999

Thera, Narada, <u>The Dhammapada: Pali Text and Translation With Stories in Brief and Notes,</u> Buddhist Cultural Centre, Dehiwela, Sri Lanka, 2000

GLOSSARY

SANSKRIT TO ENGLISH

Abhyanga....anointing, an Ayurvedic full body oil massage

Agni...fire, one of the five elements

Agnishaar...Fire Essence Breath

Akash.....the sky or ether, one of the five elements.

Analoma Viloma....Alternate Nostril Breathing

Ananda.......bliss, joy, infinite happiness

Anicca...impermanent, changing

Asana... pose or posture. Strong yet relaxed. Estimated 85,000 Yoga Asanas known

Ashram.......hermitage or monastery, place of retreat, home to all

Ashwini....Rectum pulsing

Ayama....expansion or exercise

Ayurveda...... the science or knowledge of life, *Ayurvedic* medicine is a comprehensive system of medicine, first described in the *Vedas*, based on a holistic approach rooted in earlier Vedic culture

Bhagavad Gita ....one of the great ancient Hindu scriptures, ‗Song of God'; the equivalent of the Christian New Testament to Hindus

Bhastrika.... Bellows Breath

Bhramari....Humming Bee Breath

Buddha...enlightened person

Chakra...heel, circle, vortex. Center of consciousness, 7 major ones (six on body, one above) associated with glands and nerve centers. Many minor chakras throughout body

Chandra....the moon

Chandravedi....Cooling Breath

Dharma....nature, natural law. The truth, one's destiny

Dosha.....in Ayurveda, one's constitution or nature

Dukka.....suffering, unsatisfactoriness

Dwikonasana... Fingers Laced Behind Back

Five principles of Sivananda Yoga: proper exercise (*Asanas*), proper breathing (*Pranayama*) Proper Relaxation *(Sarvasana)* Proper diet (vegetarian) positive thinking and meditation

Ghee…clarified butter, milk solids removed

Gomukhasana…Vertical Handshake

Grivasanana neck and head rolling

Guru…..teacher, one who removes darkness, brings us from dark to light

Hasta Utthanasana… Cross Hands Raised pose

Hatha…..*Ha*, the sun, the inhalation, the warm, the masculine energy. *Tha*, the moon, the exhalation, the cool, the feminine energy. Practiced together, *Hatha Yoga* and *Pranayama* banish aches, pains and illness from the body

Jai…Hail

Japa….meditation using beads

Kati Chakrasana …Seated Twist

Kapalabhati……. Shining Skull

Kundalini….divine energy, ordinarily remains dormant, at abase of spine. Goal of Yoga is to awaken and lead it to unite upward with higher Supreme consciousness

Kapha…one of the three Doshas in Ayurveda, associated with the bones, phlegm, slowness, procrastination, weight gain

Mantra…. divine sound or word from Sanskrit, devotedly repeating during meditation draws one closer to the Divine

Maranatha….I honor the God within, from the Christian Bible, Old Testament

Marjariasana…Cat Stretch

Metta…selfless love and good will

Mudra…….Yoga exercises, usually with hands, to seal or contain *Prana*

Nadi…in Ayurveda, system of channels or nerves in the human body

Namaste…….a salutation, a greeting in India for hello and goodbye. Many translations, typically the Spirit or God in me meets the God or Spirit in you. Commonly accompanied by a slight bow made with the palms touching, in front of the chest

Nauka Sanchalansana… Rowboat

Om…That alone is real, the sound of creation

Padahirasana....Cross Your Heart

Paschimottanasana ...Forward Bend

Pitta....one of the three Doshas in Ayurveda, associated with fire or heat, digestion and when disordered, inflammation and infection

Prana....... Life force, vital energy

Pranayama.......Control of *Prana*, breath. Improves concentration, uplifts spirit

Ram or Rama...one of the Hindu Gods

Rishi.......a seer or sage

Samadhi....concentration, control of one's mind

Savasana...Corpse pose

Seetkari.....Hissing Breath

Shakti...primal force that lives in humans, energy

Shanti.......peace

Sheetali.... Rolled Pipe Tongue Cooling Breath

Sri...title of respect, something like Sir

Swami.....a yogi who is the master of his senses and mind

Surya....the sun

Surya Namaskar...12 step pose, Sun Salutation

Suryavedi....Heating Breath

Swami Sivananda..... (1887-1963), considered one of the great saints of modern times, of Indian birth, a doctor prior to devoting himself to serve all

Swami Vishnudevananda....... (1927-1993) disciple of *Sivananda*, brought Yoga to Western world, established international center in Val Morin, Quebec, 1962, Sivananda Ashram Yoga Camp

Synovial fluid... A thick, clear lubricant of carbon dioxide and nitrogen found between the bones and in all joints

Tadasana and Tiryaka Tadasana...Tree and Swaying Tree poses

Trataka...Concentrated Gazing, a form of meditation

Tridosha....a balance of all three doshas or constitutions of the human body

Udjeeta...Singing *Om* in a loud pitch

Ujjayi.... Furnace Breath

Upanishads...considered the secret knowledge of gurus. Composed 1200-1300 B.C. by various writers

Utthita Lolasana ...Ragdoll

Vahipranayam... Three Locks

Vata....one of the Doshas in Ayurveda controls what is called the wind in the body, the movement like bowels, blood, breath, thoughts

Vayu.....the wind, one of the five elements

Vedas.......the original scriptures of ancient India, written about 600 B.C. contains

Vipassana....introspection, insight that totally purifies the mind

Yama....... an internal training or purification

Yoga...to yoke or unite, to join together, from the Sanskrit verb Yuj. A philosophy for living, 5000 plus years old, with eight branches of knowledge

Yogamudrasana...Psychic Union pose

Yogi, Yogini....... Practitioner of Yoga, male and female, respectively

ENGLISH TO SANSKRIT
Alternate Nostril Breathing: *Analoma Viloma*
Asana: Strong yet relaxed pose
Bellows Breath: *Bhastrika*
Bliss: *Ananda*
Calming Breath or loudly Chanting Om: *Udjeeta*
Camel: *Ustrasana*
Chopping Wood: *Kashtha Takshanasana*
Cooling Moon Breath: *Chandravedi*
Concentrated Gazing: *Trataka*
Cross Your Heart: *Padahirasana*
Crossed Hands Raised: *Hasta Utthanasana*
Expansion or exercise: *Ayama*
Fingers Laced Behind Back: Modified *Dwikonasana*
Fire Essence Breath: *Agnishaar*
Furnace Breath: *Ujjayi*
Half Butterfly: *Ardh Titali*
Head Rolling: Modified *Grivasana*
Heating Sun Breath: *Suryavedi*
Hissing Breath: *Seetkari*

Humming Bee Breath: *Bhramari*
Japa: meditation with beads
Knee Crank: *Janu Chakra*
Kneecap Contraction : *Janufalak Akarshan*
Life energy: *Prana*
Psychic Union: *Yogamudrasana*
Rectum pulsing: *Ashwini*
Roaring Lion: *Simhasana*
Rolled Pipe Tongue Cooling Breath: *Sheetali*
Seated Cat Stretch: *Marjariasana*
Seated Forward Bend: *Paschimottanasana*
Seated Rag Doll: *Utthita Lolasana*
Seated Sun Salutation: *Surya Namaskar*
Seated Tree and Swaying Tree: *Tadasana* and *Tiryaka Tadasana*
Seated Twist: Modified *Kati Chakrasana*
Shining Skull: *Kapalabhati*
Stored divine energy at the base of the spine: *Kundalini*
Three Locks: *Vahipranayam*
Vertical Handshake: *Gomukhasana*

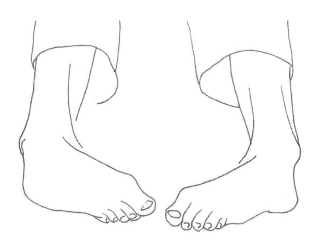

Made in the USA
Columbia, SC
10 November 2023

25856312R00102